Praise for Empo~~wered Birth~~

Being a sport psychologist while becoming a mother has been one of the greatest experiences of my life. I am confident that what I have learned and practiced in my professional role has enhanced my own journey of becoming a mother and I'm thrilled that Carla has decided to share with others the powerful lessons and skills that sport psychology can offer in this space. I know that these skills have the potential to make a very positive impact on new moms!

Dr Chelsi Day, Clinical Sport Psychologist and Certified Mental Performance Coach

As a sport and exercise psychologist, I have long been fascinated by the role the mind plays in sport. Having then applied many a mental strategy during both of my home births, I am also a huge advocate of educating parents-to-be about the role their mind can play before, during and after labour, and helping them to use it effectively. "Empowered birth" is a readable, practical book, filled with useful tips and techniques for you to discover and use throughout your labour and beyond!

Juliette Lloyd, Mother and Sport Psychologist

This is a book I wish I could have read prior to my experience of becoming a mother. As a physiologist I know little about the ways that Psychology could have helped me through these experiences. This book will provide valuable detail for those about to embark on the journey of motherhood.

Dr Jessica Hill, Associate Professor in Physiology at St Mary's University

As an exercise psychologist, researcher of physical activity during the perinatal period, and an active mother myself, I am an advocate of learning from the sport and exercise field and applying the knowledge to the maternity journey. From our research we now further understand the challenges and benefits of engaging with physical activity during this time. Psychological techniques that are fine-tuned during physical activity behaviour, such as self-talk to cheer yourself on, or learning to set process goals, can benefit those who are keen to stay active throughout their pregnancy, and these can be drawn on during labour and beyond.

Dr Hayley Mills, Chartered Sport and Exercise Psychologist, Director of Perinatal Physical Activity Research Group, Chair of the expert group commissioned by the UK Chief Medical Officers (CMO) for the development of the Postpartum Physical Activity Guidelines.

Empowered Birth helps women to find and fully feel their natural strength. Dr Meijen helps mothers to understand that endurance is an internal resource, that exists within them, waiting to be tapped. This book is inspiring and reassuring in equal measure.

Natalie Meddings, doula and author of How to Have a Baby

Like many expectant mothers I made a birthing plan... which during labour then turned into fiction! By practicing what I preach as an applied sport psychologist I was able to maintain a sense of calm determination and enjoy the experience. This book, the first of its kind, is well worth a read in considering how to apply psychological strategies for the benefit of your own birthing experience.

Professor Tracey Devonport, University of Wolverhampton

I have pushed myself in sports from a very young age, so when it came to preparing for birth, I knew that the strength and mental energy techniques that had become second nature to me, would help me with the physical challenges of pregnancy and birth. When my first birth resulted in an emergency C-section in the middle of labour, rather than letting the situation overwhelm me, I found it easy to adapt to the new situation. On the way the operating theatre, breathing and visualisation techniques helped me feel calm during the intense pain of contractions. Being in a calm state helped my body cope. The positive mental attitude I learnt from competitive sports certainly helped me cope with the challenges of childbirth. Everyone can benefit from the strength, wellbeing and positive thinking honed by (endurance) sports, especially during childbirth.

Melissa Hogenboom, Author of
The Motherhood Complex

Pregnancy, childbirth and parenthood is a journey in life that can be both amazing and overwhelming. Often the societal narrative and expectations are set out in such a way that pain and exhaustion can seem inevitable. Carla uses her expertise to skilfully demonstrate that the way we enable our bodies and minds to work together in harmony through sport can be applied effectively to the childbearing journey by conceptualising it as a physical and emotional journey with which we have our own individual relationship, ability to plan and make our own. The extraordinary thing for me as a psychiatrist, rugby player and coach is how our skills as parents can be applied back to sport, for example, as more receptive and nurturing coaches and more effective team players.

Dr Rebecca Syed Sheriff, Consultant Psychiatrist and Senior
Clinical Research Fellow

I whole heartedly agree with using what you know from your days as an athlete, or learning skills from the mindset of an athlete, is a good set of tools to have as you prepare for and go through labor, childbirth and during postpartum. Focusing on what is right in front of you, staying in the moment, a positive, flexible mindset, deep breathing and how to use breathing for strength and remaining calm were all skills I used during my maternity journey that I learned in my days as a competitive and professional ice skater.

Lynette Damir, Registered Nurse, Founder of SwaddleDesigns

I can definitely see similarities between sport psychology and pregnancy/motherhood. During my pregnancy I took care of my body like an athlete. I listened to my body what it needed at that moment, and before giving birth I made sure all of my preparations were done, and I made time for myself to get ready for 'my game'. I have never been that determined and confident about myself and I had trust in the people around me while giving birth. Visualizing waves of the sea helped me to deal with contractions. Although I was induced, labour went quite easy. I still believe that taking care of body and mind (I've worked on body awareness and coped with a lot of different emotions) helped me to facilitate labour. Once my son was born I've spent a lot of time alone with him. I took my time to recover while keeping calm by slow breathing so my heartrate would go down in order to connect with my baby. I can definitely say I relied on myself and was 'in the flow'.

Justine Loosveldt, Sport and Exercise Psychologist and Clinical Psychologist

As someone who is a practicing Sport Psychologist teaching mental skills to athletes every day I am disappointed I never thought to use these skills when I went on my own maternity journey to become a mum as it makes such perfect sense to do so. Dr Meijen has entwined the benefits of sport psychology beautifully with the challenges of maternity to show how we can use the strengths-based processes we use daily with athletes to make that time when women are pregnant and birthing far easier, more enjoyable and with that important feeling of being more in control.

Dr Josephine Perry, Sport Psychologist and author of I Can: The Teenage Athlete's Guide to Mental Fitness

Empowered Birth: Lessons from Sport Psychology for Your Maternity Journey

Every possible effort has been made to ensure that the information contained in this book is accurate at the time of going to press. The publishers and author(s) cannot accept responsibility for any errors and omissions, however caused. No responsibility for loss or damage occasioned to any person acting, or refraining from action, as a result of the material contained in this publication can be accepted by the editor, the publisher or the author.

First published in 2023 by Sequoia Books

ISBN
Print: 9781914110245
EPUB: 9781914110252

A CIP record for this book is available from the British Library

Library of Congress Cataloguing-In-Publication Data

Name: Carla Meijen
Title: Empowered Birth/Carla Meijen
Description: 1st Edition, Sequoia Books UK 2023
Subjects: RG: Pregnancy
Print: 9781914110245
EPUB: 9781914110252

Library of Congress Control Number: 2023906241

Print and Electronic production managed by Deanta Global

Empowered Birth: Lessons from Sport Psychology for Your Maternity Journey

by
Dr. Carla Meijen

SEQUOIA
B O O K S

Contents

Acknowledgements and thanks

Thinking back, the idea for this book was planted during my pregnancy yoga classes. The teacher was genuinely interested in the women who attended her classes, and she ensured to draw on their skills and strengths in the class. It made me aware how powerful sport and my background in sport psychology could be in helping me to prepare for giving birth. In the months after giving birth while I was talking to other women about our birth stories I realised how useful the techniques that I teach to sports people and students were during the different stages of labour. When I then discovered that there was no such resource the idea of writing a book on what we can learn from sport psychology during the maternity journey was born.

It could have easily stayed just an idea, were it not from the encouragement from my partner and friends. I wrote a book proposal, which Aly Ribis who worked as a midwife at the time, reviewed. Her positive review was the confidence boost I needed. Thank you to Andy Peart and Sequoia Books for taking on the idea, and for your suggestions and support throughout the process.

As part of the book, I interviewed women about their birth story, and I asked them about the impact that their background in sport had when giving birth. I thoroughly loved listening to the stories of all these amazing women, and I am so grateful for their openness when sharing their birth stories. Here is a big thank you to Chrissie Wellington, Paola Bisi, Chemmy Alcott, Imke Veltman, Sabine van Elsland, Amy Williams, Pip Davies, Alda Wong, Jo Vidal, Emma During, Funmi Olatoye, and Joy Black.

A big thank you to Danielle Adams. Thank you for talking me through the decompression stages and how you have implemented these in your work. Most importantly, thank you for listening and supporting me. Thank you to Kelly Massey for talking to me about your research on pregnancy and motherhood in elite sport, such a fascinating research area! It was a little daunting to ask people to proofread chapters, thank you so much for this Jo Vidal, Alda Wong, Emily Martin, and Martin Turner.

Thanks to mama, papa, and Rick. Growing up in a physically active family in the Netherlands fuelled my love for sports. I was always so proud of my mum when she came back after long cycle rides in the weekends, I watched my dad play table tennis, and I remember how much I enjoyed cycling next to him on my little bicycle when he went out for a run, and my brother got me into playing basketball which I can't thank him enough for.

The biggest thank you of all goes to Erik, you mean so much to me and your support has been so important for me to write this book. Tack så jätte mycket. And to Robyn, you are my inspiration and without you I would not have written this book. I love you both to the moon and back.

1   Ready, steady … Sport psychology and your maternity journey

"At the Olympics, you are scared, you have fear, you are really nervous, you have got all of this anxiety and negative feelings before a race. I would always flip it into 'I am not scared, I am just excited'. 'I am not nervous, I am just ready'. So, I already flipped that self-talk in very positive things, and so for me, it was like, I am going to do the same. I am excited to give birth and I am excited to know what it feels like. It is a new thing I have never done before and I am excited to hold my baby. That really helped". Amy Williams (skeleton, Olympic gold medallist)

The maternity journey is often compared to a marathon, a long journey that requires grit, endurance, pacing and patience, dealing with pain and discomfort, and motivation to stay on track. As a sport psychologist I work with endurance athletes, and as an academic I research the psychological aspects of endurance performance. When I was on my pregnancy journey, I found it striking how many similarities there are between giving birth and endurance activities. Not only when it comes to the mental qualities of pulling yourself through that marathon but also how you can manage the psychological demands of endurance events. When I was pregnant, I kept thinking, 'how can I use my experience working in sport psychology when it comes to coping with giving birth?' Hearing the stories from others who were pregnant or who had recently given birth made me come back to this question. This book is very much inspired by conversations with mothers where it became evident to me how the sporting experiences of women can be so empowering and helpful during the maternity journey, and the idea of writing this book was born.

In this book, I share how sport psychology can be applied to the maternity journey. I set out how mothers-to-be can use mental strategies commonly adopted by people in sport to focus on their strengths to see the birthing experience as a positive challenge. Doing sport can be a great vehicle to practice one's mental strength. Throughout the book I give information about sport psychology and how athletes use sport psychology, with practical tips on how mental strategies can be used in a range of situations. What I hope you will take away from this book is that you feel empowered by what is already available to you, and maybe you will learn and take on board a new strategy or two that can help you manage the challenges of your maternity journey. If you can use these strategies after giving birth, all the better!

What's important to clarify at the outset of the book is that I am a qualified sport and exercise psychologist, and the focus of the book is on sharing my knowledge and application of sport psychology. I am not a medical expert, and therefore I am not someone who is positioned to advice on the medical aspects of pregnancy and childbirth. If you are intending to practice any of the sport psychology strategies *during* sport and exercise activities whilst you are pregnant, it is useful to speak to a trained expert to understand what you can and cannot do in terms of physical activity. I am a big advocate of promoting staying active during your maternity journey if the situation allows it, and you may find that there may be some opportunities for you to strengthen and practice mental strategies whilst doing sport and exercise.

Women in sport

There is an impressive list of athletes who have either competed whilst pregnant or returned to their sport after giving birth to accomplish impressive feats. Tennis players Kim Clijsters and Serena Williams won grand slams, endurance athlete Jo Pavey won the 10000 meter European Championships, sprinter Alysson Felix won a gold medal at the world championships less than a year after giving birth, 800 meter runner Alysia Montano ran a race when heavily pregnant, cyclist Sarah Storey set multiple world records after having a baby, equestrian Anky van Grunsven won multiple Olympic medals in dressage, basketball players Candace Parker and Lisa Leslie both won the WNBA championship as mums, and ultra-runner Sophie Power breastfed her three-month-old son during the 103-mile (165 km) Ultra du Mont Blanc. This is just a small list of athletes, and it does not include all the amazing mothers and mothers-to-be who are not in the spotlight. I believe this latter point is so important to emphasise; we hear and read the stories of elite and well-known women who often have the support around them to be able to train during pregnancy and return to sport. There are, however, so many stories of women who exercise or play sports and do this whilst also having a job or looking after their children. These stories are just as empowering. And you may be one of these amazing women!

Much of the focus of stories about pregnant athletes has been on their physical and physiological ability to return to high-performance sports. Some of these stories have highlighted how giving birth has helped women to change their perspective as an athlete, whether this is how they experience pain, or whether they not just see themselves as an athlete, but as a mother. After giving birth for the first time, often a new identity is born too, that of a mother. It is very common for someone whose life has been dominated by sports to feel that most of their identity comes from being an athlete and their involvement in sport. When they give birth, they suddenly become a mother too, and a different identity needs to be established to accommodate this new role. This consideration of how your identity could change is really important to consider, but I will park this for now until the final chapter of this book.

The stories of women who won sporting events when pregnant or when returning to their sport after giving birth can be both fascinating and inspirational stories to read and learn from, yet equally inspiring is how experiences of women in sport have helped them to mentally prepare for giving birth and managing pain. The world of sport is intriguing, and there is so much we can take away and learn from sport. When we consider sport performance, this includes physical, physiological, tactical, technical, as well as mental qualities. There is also the support network, such as the sporting organisation, coaches, teammates, and so on. The interaction between all of these is helpful to keep in mind, because although the focus of this book is on sport psychology, you need to have at least an awareness of the interplay of all these aspects to understand and help to get the most out of sport performance.

So what? What is the role of sport psychology in all of this?

There are so many ways of doing sport psychology, such as focusing on the systems someone is functioning in, taking a person-centred approach, to embrace personal freedom and personal growth, or to adopt a cognitive-behavioural approach, just to name a few. A popular approach in sport psychology, and psychology in general, is that what we think influences how we feel and what we do. Our thoughts, feelings, and behaviour are related. Let's give you an example – you may be working out in the gym and doing some strength exercises you have not done before. If you think, 'This is tough, I am not strong enough for this' (thoughts), you may feel deflated or insecure (feelings) and stop trying (behaviour). Or perhaps you think, 'This is a bit different than what I have done before, let's see what it's like' (thoughts), you may feel excited (feelings), and give it another go when you lose your balance (behaviour). My take on this is that we can try to influence and use our thoughts, either by actively changing them or by trying to pay close attention to them, observing them, and seeing thoughts for what they are. This latter point is important, as you simply cannot change every single thought that comes in your brain – you'd be exhausted! And when you are paying close attention to your thoughts and observing them, you may also start to notice helpful thoughts. This can be really empowering, as you can start to learn to tune in to these helpful (and often positive) thoughts. At various stages in the book, I will explain how you can use psychological techniques, such as self-talk, imagery, and mindfulness-based strategies, to help manage thoughts and feelings.

A misconception that some people have of sport psychology is that sport psychologists focus on 'fixing' something that is wrong. Of course, as a sport psychologist, there have been times where I have worked with sports people to help address difficulties they may encounter, and working with sports people and their mental health is also common in sports. Notably, well-being is typically at the forefront of the work of a sport psychologist. But this does not necessarily mean that it is about 'fixing' something that is wrong. What I like to draw your attention to is that sport psychology can be just as much about building on your strengths rather than feeling stuck focusing on and trying to fix your weaknesses. As human beings, we are naturally more tuned in to our negative experiences than to our positive experiences. This serves a function, such as protecting us and helping to avoid harm, but it is not always useful. What I try to achieve through a strength-based approach is to help people be more tuned into their positive experiences, and to reflect and build on their strengths, rather than constantly trying to 'fix' something that they feel is wrong or trying really hard to avoid their weaknesses. I strongly believe that this can be a powerful approach to help you prepare for labour too. I am not saying it will be easy to suddenly make a radical shift towards only focusing on the positives, and there is a space and time for reflecting on negative or less helpful experiences too. If you know you are someone who tends to tune in much more to the negatives than the positives, then here is an exercise you can try to start becoming more aware of your strengths.

After your next sport or exercise session, take a few minutes to reflect on the positives of the activity. If you do not have any exercise or sport activities planned, maybe because you are not in a position to do so, you can think back about a competition you played in, or a race you competed in, that was meaningful to you, or a hard gym session. Alternatively, you can reflect on an important meeting or presentation. Once you have an activity or situation in mind, answer the following questions:

1. What was the experience?
2. What went through your mind?
3. What did you feel?
4. What did you do that may have played a role in this?
5. What went well?
6. What have you learned from the experience?

Doing reflective tasks is not easy, especially if you are not used to it, and it takes a few goes to get familiar doing it. A strength-based approach can be helpful because most people will have used some kind of strategy to overcome or manage demanding situations, in the sporting arena or in the workplace, but we often overlook or forget about these. Doing reflective tasks can help you to become much more aware of the bank of experiences that you have already built, and it can feel encouraging to know that you have already got some tools in the toolbox to deal with potentially difficult or demanding situations. This is relevant, because there may not always be scope to learn a lot of new strategies in the lead-up to birth. Rather, focusing on strengthening what is already available can be a more efficient use of your time and energy. Joy Black, a rock climber and personal trainer, explained that when she is rock climbing, she decides which hold to use – the safety assessments are her responsibility – and doing this makes her feel strong as a 'bad-ass'. She would not let anyone tell her that she 'couldn't climb above that'. In the lead-up to the birth of her third child, she asked herself, 'Why can't I use this confidence and assertiveness during labour'? Reflecting on how mentally and physically strong she is as a rock climber made her feel empowered, and she realised that she can be powerful and transfer these skills to labour. This confidence and assertiveness that can come with doing competitive sports and hard workouts are worth taking on board with you.

The purpose of this book is not to advocate that you should be a warrior. That is not what a strength-based approach is about. This approach of feeling you need to be a warrior can set a dangerous precedent and affect mental health. Also, remember that just because you are physically strong as an athlete, this does not mean that you will automatically have an easy birth and that is okay. Where traditionally a lot of focus in sport is on performance, athletes have started to open up about their mental health in recent years. At Olympic Games in the past, it was often about celebrating the exceptional performances of sports people and praising them for their win-at-all-cost mentality. We only need to think about the praise the American gymnast Kerri Strug received when she performed the vault on a broken ankle to win team gold at the 1996 Olympic Games. This perform-at-all-costs mind-set seemed to have shifted somewhat at the Tokyo 2020 Olympics; these Olympic Games appeared to be the first big multi-sport event where sportspeople were more willing to share their concerns about their mental health openly. Simone Biles, also an American gymnast, withdrew from the team event because of mental health reasons. This openness is such an important step, and the emphasis on mental health during the pandemic may have helped to contribute to this narrative. What I would like to state is that concerns around mental health have been prevalent for many years, but sportspeople have often not felt comfortable sharing their concerns openly and publicly. When it comes to sport psychology, traditionally there has been a big focus on high-performance and elite sports; there is now more of an appreciation that sport psychology can benefit people from all levels of sport. This is important to remember, as a lot of what I talk about in the book applies to people playing sports at all levels.

Let's pick up on stress and worries for a moment here. A strength of sport psychology as a discipline is that it draws from other domains in psychology and sport, such as physiology and biological psychology, to help understand behaviour of those involved in sport and exercise.

When it comes to stress and worries, this is very relevant to emphasise as our body works as a unit. For example, if we feel under pressure and start to feel stressed, this has an influence on the hormone interactions in our body. In particular, stress can lead to increases in a hormone called cortisol. Cortisol can be helpful in that it can give a spike in energy (helpful when you need some extra energy to push the baby out!), but too much of it can be unhelpful. Continuous spikes in cortisol tend to wear us out. Experiencing stress and pain also releases beta-endorphins which help relieve pain. Beta-endorphins are also produced when you exercise, have sex or laugh. These endorphins are useful as it helps to relieve pain, and as such endorphins can be 'your friend' in those tough sport workouts and in labour, but excessive stress and subsequent high beta-endorphin levels can inhibit oxytocin (sometimes called the 'love' hormone, which helps to stimulate contractions) and slow labour down. In summary, a hormone equilibrium (in the popular media sometimes referred to as 'balance') is helpful during labour to help get your body ready, initiate and keep contractions going, and also to help prepare your body and the baby for what's about to come. Too much stress and worries can disrupt this equilibrium. Having this awareness that our body works as a unit can be helpful to work out what may disrupt the equilibrium.

A comparison some could resonate with to understand the impact of stress is to compare it to an engine. For example, imagine you are running late for an important appointment and feel worried about it. You have decided to drive to the appointment, and rather than driving calmly, you are constantly changing speed to overtake other cars to try to get to your destination as quickly as possible, without much luck as you are having to stop at all the red lights on the way. If you constantly change speed, then you'll be using a lot more fuel, you might even run out of fuel because you have no time to fill up the car and you increase the wear and tear on the car engine. This may also happen in sport situations. Let's take a marathon, you are aiming to get a particular time to qualify for another event, and lots of people you know are watching, which is making you feel really stressed. With your thoughts all over the place, you forget your race plan, get out of the 'start blocks' too fast, don't take enough fluids during the early stages of the race, and are running out of energy well before the finish line. When you are in labour, you don't want to feel like you are running late for an appointment or expand all your energy at the start. An ideal setting is one where there is a hormone equilibrium which is often in a calm setting, without too many disruptions.

I will talk more about stress in chapters 2 and 3. What is useful when trying to create a calm setting is to think about some of the things that ramp up your stress levels. For example, one of the factors that can increase stress in the lead-up and during labour are concerns about pain. It is difficult to disregard the word 'pain' when it comes to giving birth, and it is quite likely that there will be some element of pain during and/or after, when you recover from giving birth or from the caesarean section surgery. Women I spoke with, from Olympians, climbers, to cross-fit athletes, explained that labour pain was like no other pain they had ever experienced, and for some of them the pain was completely overwhelming. Others experienced the pain as intense but were able to manage it, saw it as part of the process, and, even though very different as a type of pain, they felt that the intensity was not dissimilar to sport injuries they had incurred. Labour pain is complex; there are so many physiological, physical, and psychological processes that interact. This makes it that the pain experience is a sub-jective and very individual experience. Interestingly, the combination of hormones during labour also plays a role in how we remember the pain that we experienced in the moment. Perhaps this is why some-times, even though labour has been a rather painful experience in that moment, women don't remember the pain as that intense which can help them to remember giving birth as a positive experience. Similar findings have been reported when it comes to remembering the inten-sity of the pain after running a marathon too!

One thing that can be really difficult is to try to change the rela-tionship you have with pain when in labour, to work with it and not against it. Where pain in sport often signals that something is wrong, pain during labour serves a different purpose. In addition, in sports, and endurance sports in particular, the decision to expose yourself to pain and discomfort can be a volitional decision. You know that those long runs or swims will hurt. That is, you made a choice to expose yourself to the pain. You can stop doing the activity or take a break when the pain becomes too much or signals that something is wrong such as an injury. During labour, pain is often inevitable; it is not as if you can suddenly stop a contraction. Pain in labour serves a function; in fact, it is part of the process to get the baby out! Pain is therefore not always a warning sign that something is wrong, and being afraid of the pain might trigger you to go into fight-or-flight mode or 'attack' mode. This can be quite unhelpful as your focus will be moved away from the process of giving birth (I will come back to this in chapter 8)! Labour can be painful, and as I mentioned already, for some women, it is like no other pain they have experienced. But, you can learn to adapt how you approach the labour pain and embrace the pain rather than try-ing to fight against it. Chemmy Alcott (Alpine skiing; Olympian) told me that once she changed her relationship with pain and embraced it, she started to enjoy it as she understood what the purpose of the pain was. Tuning in to the pain may also help you to become aware of when the pain does not feel 'right', which is important to discuss with your medical team, as some types of pain can indicate that something is amiss. Throughout the book, I will cover different techniques of how to manage pain; this includes examples of how you could change how you see pain, the role of breathing, control and learning to let go. Before this, let's briefly cover the basics of pain as a concept.

Pain is such a fascinating concept and entire books have been writ-ten about it. I will only cover some of the very basic aspects here. When we talk about pain, it can be helpful to distinguish between pain tolerance, pain threshold, and pain intensity. Pain tolerance is simply said to be the amount of pain you are able to tolerate until it becomes too much. A very popular task in psychology research is the cold pressor task, where people are asked to put a hand in a bucket of very cold (ice) water. Their pain threshold is reached when they first experience pain after putting their hand in the bucket of water. Pain tolerance is then measured by how long they are keeping their hand in the water before pulling the hand out. Then there is also the intensity of the pain, which is about the magnitude of the pain. It's helpful to know the difference between pain threshold, pain tolerance, and pain intensity. Perhaps your pain threshold and tolerance are quite high, but during labour the pain intensity is very high, a 9 or 10 out of 10. Maybe you experience six contractions or more in a ten-minute period, where you have barely got any time to recover in between contractions. I interviewed a few Dutch women, and the Dutch have an appropriate word for this: 'weeënstorm', which translates to a storm, or tornado, of contractions. For some people, this pain intensity can become too much to bear, even though they may have a high pain threshold and pain tolerance. For others, the pain intensity is manageable, maybe because they have released appropriate amounts of beta-endorphins. Just relying on your pain threshold without considering intensity levels can lead to some unhelpful thoughts and feelings. Similarly, you may be positively surprised with how you are experiencing the pain. It is also helpful to understand that pain intensity changes throughout labour, and awareness of the different phases of labour can help you prepare your pain management strategies. It is a bit like a marathon, where you will be drawing on different psychological strategies throughout the event to manage pain and discomfort.

What happens in the phases of labour? Very simply said, contractions typically move from Braxton Hicks (practice contractions) to early labour, active labour, transition, to pushing. Transition contractions are quite different from early labour and initial active labour. It may be a relatively short phase, but transition contractions are intense, with shorter breaks and a lot of physical pressure on the vagina and rectum. A lot of concentration and energy is required for this stage as you feel the need to push, but typically the body is not quite ready for this if the cervix is not fully dilated. It is helpful to think about the different demands in these phases, because a different strategy may be required to help manage the pain. It may be that visualisation strategies work well during early and active labour, but if it becomes too much when the pain becomes all-encompassing at the transition stage, you may find that you draw more on breathing strategies.

If you want to know more about the details of these stages, I recommend that you do some reading about the stages of labour to help you feel prepared, attend an antenatal course, or speak to a health professional. To share my experience, all I remember from my birth classes was the emphasis on differentiating between early and active labour to make sure you wouldn't go to or contact the hospital too quickly. I did not really consider the different (mental) demands of the phases. I just had this thought that contractions are painful but had not consciously considered adapting my strategies across the stages of labour. I believe that mentally preparing for these phases and the changes in the pain intensity are helpful in making informed decisions when it comes to aspects such as pain relief. The great thing is that there is a lot of information available to equip yourself with. Just make sure that you check the source of information, and if you are attending antenatal classes, you check the qualifications of the educator. It is fascinating how much variance there is in the information on delivering a baby and how this can inform our decision-making and confidence in our ability to manage pain. When you are experiencing pain in the moment, it is probably not the time to learn about these different stages! My take-home message here is to do some homework to help you prepare and feel calm.

How you want to approach pain during the birthing experience is such a personal thing; it is important that you go with what feels right for you. If you do not want to experience more pain than is necessary, go for it. If you want to have a home birth where you don't have access to an epidural, and it's possible for you to do so, go for it. Do what feels right for you, and don't feel you need to be a warrior fighting through pain if that does not sit well with you. How we experience pain is very personal, and I would urge you not to compare yourself to others or feel pressured into making decisions that you feel uncomfortable with. Not only is this unhelpful, but it can give you a lot of unnecessary stress and worries, which is not ideal when you try to create a calm environment!

How to use the book?

The maternity journey and giving birth are incredibly personal and every woman will bring their own experiences to this. Therefore, there is no 'one size, fits all' approach to best manage the maternity journey. What I would love for you to take away from this book is to learn about how you can use different sport psychology-inspired strategies during your journey so that you have the ingredients to prepare your own 'soup' of strategies. You may not need all of them or feel that you have the time and opportunity to practice all the different strategies. It's a bit like cooking, where you may have to adapt the recipe based on what you have in your cupboard and as such the result may not always be the same, but it still works. None of the strategies are revolutionary or groundbreaking; some of them originate from other domains, such as health, education, and clinical psychology, and some of the strategies are regularly used during childbirth already. A lot of women are, however, not aware that they are already quite good at using some of these strategies and fail to make the link between different areas of their life, such as a sport, the workplace, and childbirth. It is helpful to sometimes think a bit outside of the box, which is what I have tried to do with this book by focusing on what you have learned from playing sport and doing exercise. I find it surprising how often we forget to transfer skills we got from one part of our life to other parts.

In the book, I will start with setting out how you can see the birthing experience as a positive challenge and not as a negative threat. Drawing on research, I explain what the components are that contribute to transforming a demanding situation in a challenge; these include self-belief, feeling you are in control, and tackling the situation 'head on'. In chapter 3, I will go into the emotional rollercoaster that the birthing experience can be for some. I will outline where emotions come from and start introducing some ways of managing, but not suppressing, emotions. Chapters 4, 5, 6, 7, and 8 set out strategies that can help you approach the birthing experience as a positive challenge. Chapter 9 emphasises the importance of drawing on your environment and provides suggestions on how you can use social support. The final chapter is about 'bringing it home', and some considerations on how the psychological strategies could be useful in the post-partum period.

As I go through the strategies, you may notice that these are linked and that there is at times an overlap between the strategies. It does feel a little bit artificial to divide these up into separate chapters, but for the sake of simplicity, this is what I have done, as otherwise, the book may end up being a little bit much to digest. With these strategies, it is important that you allow yourself some time to practice them. This may be during an exercise or yoga session, where you may try out different self-talk statements, imagery, focusing techniques, or breathing. Throughout the book, there will be some tasks that are intended to assist you with this. Even when you may not feel you have the time to practice, you can reflect on what you are already using and consider how you can adapt this to a labour setting.

Reflection is key to something called self-regulation. Our behaviour tends to be driven by goals, and self-regulation is about those processes that guide you towards or away from goals. This can be through trying to manage your thoughts, feelings, and behaviour in a way that will help you in the pursuit of that goal. In practical terms, it could be the amount of effort you are willing to put into a task or to use a relaxation strategy to calm down in the heat of a moment. It is helpful to know about self-regulation because this can benefit how we get to where we would like to be.

How can you self-regulate? One approach is self-regulated learning, which is a cyclical process with three phases – the forethought phase, the performance phase, and the self-reflection phase. In the forethought phase, you consider the task that needs to be done, set goals for these, and plan. People high in self-regulation tend to set specific process and outcome goals (more about this in chapter 4), often use technique-oriented strategies, and have high levels of self-belief.

The performance phase is about 'doing', where you do the task, consider how you are doing in relation to the task, and draw on strategies such as imagery (more about this in chapter 5), engaging your support system, time management, and so on, to help achieve the task. Finally, the reflection phase is about assessing how the task went, what were the reasons it went well or did not go so well? Often thinking about why it went well or not so well makes us feel happy, sad, or another emotion. This can then inform how we look at the task in the future; it also informs our self-belief for the next time we engage in the task and when we are in the forethought phase again.

I appreciate that this may feel abstract; the key take-home message is that without this self-reflection phase, you might get stuck in doing the same thing over and over again or get frustrated without really understanding why or how to manage this differently going forward. In the last chapter of this book, we will get back to reflection.

To finish this chapter, there are five points that I hope you find useful to keep in mind as you are making your way through this book. These are:

1. **Practice**

    Give yourself an opportunity to put the different strategies into practice. Having practiced the strategies will make you feel more confident that you know how they work; it will also give you an insight into which strategies you want to have in your toolbox. Moreover, having already thought about when you may be using the strategies gives you easier access to them when you feel overwhelmed.

2. **Control the controllables, let go of the uncontrollable**

    Giving birth can feel like it has quite a few unpredictable events, as does the maternity journey. This is okay. Think about what is within your control and what is not. Adapt and adjust where feasible, but also realise that sometimes you do not need to change anything, and patience and perhaps drawing in support is what is needed.

3. **Prepare as you would for a marathon**

   You don't prepare for a marathon overnight. You can replicate the planning and investment that come with sport or other areas of your lives when it comes to preparing for giving birth. How can you look after yourself, what can you do in terms of planning, rest and recovery? Empower yourself with information and identify reputable resources to help you.

4. **Be kind to yourself**

   Pregnancy and labour are intense enough as it is already. Your body is changing, and the fluctuations in hormones can also have a big impact. If you can't quite get as much done in a day or something does not work out, that's okay.

5. **Don't feel that you need to do everything by yourself**

   Ensure to seek advice if needed, and don't push through when it does not feel right. You are the expert on your body; you know your body best.

2 Seeing the maternity journey as a positive challenge, not a threat

Ask yourself a question – how do you feel about giving birth, do you see it as a positive challenge (an opportunity) or as a threat? Take a minute or two to think about this. Next, write down a few words that you associate with giving birth as an opportunity, and do the same for words you associate with feeling that giving birth is a threat.

Before venturing into doing research on the psychology of endurance performance, I completed a PhD on challenge and threat states in athletes. Simply said, in this research, I look at how sportspeople feel about competition where there is lots at stake. Do they see it as a challenge (in this context, as something positive, an opportunity) or as a threat? We propose that those who see it as a positive challenge feel they have more control over the situation, have more self-belief, take an active approach to deal with the situation, and feel that their emotional state is generally helpful. The way their body deals with the demanding situation is more beneficial, their blood flow increases, and their vascular resistance reduces. More recently, we have also proposed that there is more oxytocin in a challenge state. All of this is relevant when it comes to giving birth.

Control

Let's start with control. A lot of time we want to take control over a lot of things around us, and giving birth is no different. We think we have control over what's going to happen, and writing a detailed birth plan is a prime example of this. If you speak to mothers who have given birth and ask how much they were able to stick with their birth plan, you are probably told that the birth plan, or part of it at least, went out of the window. Perhaps the baby decided to turn last minute, the baby's heart rate dropped, after your waters have broken the baby desperately needed to poo before coming out into the big world or it all just went a little bit quicker than expected and you were stronger than giving yourself credit for beforehand. Letting go of the birth plan can be tough, as it feels that you are letting go of control. Ask yourself the question – Is it really that bad to let go of trying to control every aspect? When you think about it, trying to over-control is not helpful – especially not in labour when too much adrenaline and cortisol can interfere with contractions and feeling relaxed. So, knowing that wanting to be in control is not that helpful when it comes to giving birth, why do I suggest that it can help you to approach birth as a positive challenge and not as a threat?

Let me explain, the feeling of having control is not the same as being in control or wanting to be in control. What you want to focus on is what you perceive to have control over, which is 'subjective' control. It's about focusing on 'controlling the controllables', which is a common saying in sports and an expression used by a few of the women I interviewed. It is not about objective control or what outsiders feel you can control, or trying to control external factors. In sporting settings, I often use the weather as an example. It is pretty difficult to control the weather, but what you can control is what you wear or how you mentally will deal with the weather. For example, if you are running in the rain, you can wear a rain jacket and shoes with more grip. If you are playing tennis in windy weather conditions, you can adapt your game plan based on the side of the court you are playing. If it is cold before your football match, you can ensure that you are properly dressed and adjust your warm-up. Dealing with unexpected weather conditions is not always that easy, but accepting that the weather is a factor you cannot control nor change is already a helpful step. When we translate this to giving birth, you cannot always control which room or hospital you give birth in, whether you will have a water birth or not, or how the baby will respond throughout the different stages of labour. There are some aspects that you can control, for example, you may be able to bring music with you that makes it feel more comfortable or bring essential oils, like peppermint or lavender with you if that's something that would work for you. Let's also not forget all the psychological strategies that you can bring with you! Maybe your motivational mantras, breathing techniques, visualisation/imagery and so on. We will cover a range of these later in the book.

To help you with this idea of control, here is a task you can try. This task is a self-reflection and self-awareness exercise. If you have a birth plan, or have started to think about your birth plan, make a list of the different components that make up your birth plan. For example, movement during labour, having music, choice of midwife, birth centre, epidural, C-section, and so on. Write down next to each one whether you feel that each aspect is within your control or not.

The birth plan is an important part of preparing for labour, but at the same time it is important to prepare for the unexpected. Now you have thought about the different types of control, you can start thinking about how you could let go of control or alter parts of the birth plan. Giving away control can be hard unless you are prepared for it. Therefore, what I would also recommend is to think about how it might make you feel when you would have to make these changes. Preparing for this in advance can be a helpful coping strategy. I talk more about this in the chapters about if-then planning and goal setting (chapter 4) and emotion management (chapter 3).

Self-belief

Self-efficacy, or self-belief, is important too. Self-efficacy is about what we believe we can do, it is not about our intention (what you believe you will do) or experience (what you have done). An example is having the belief in yourself that you can push through pain, which is different from having the thought that you think you will push through the pain. Both of these can be useful, but for now I want to focus on the first (I believe I can) as there are a lot of positive and helpful outcomes related to this. The tricky thing about self-efficacy is that it can change quickly based on the information that is available to you and it can be fragile especially after negative feedback. One moment you believe you can push through the pain, and before you know it, the belief has faded, perhaps because the midwife has told you that you are 'only' a few centimetres dilated, a new person enters the room, or your partner tells you that you look tired. Feeling self-efficacious can be helpful when you face obstacles or a difficult situation.

Knowing that self-efficacy can be helpful and important, how can you increase your self-belief, and perhaps equally important, how do you make it 'robust', so that it is less impacted by negative feedback or experiences? To do so, it is helpful to understand that self-efficacy can be broken down into different 'sources', that is, self-efficacy is a combination of previous performance accomplishments, role models (vicarious experiences), verbal persuasion, physiological arousal (effort perception), imaginal experiences, and emotional arousal.

If this is the first time you will be going into labour, then drawing on previous childbirth experiences is something that may not be available to you. Having experienced labour previously is not the only experience that could inform your belief in your ability to manage the labour experience. For example, you can draw on times where you experienced how strong your body is. There are plenty of relevant experiences, such as instances where you had to push through pain or discomfort, had to fight through fatigue, or when you found another gear when running out of energy. You can look at this as the power of recollection, where you think back about instances where you know you had to overcome pain or discomfort, find another level of energy, or put your body in a position that can be helpful, such as squatting. Knowing that a contraction typically lasts one minute is also helpful to keep in mind, for example – are you able to do an activity such as triceps dips or squatting for one minute? Having the experience that you can manage this even when it feels uncomfortable, can also help to give you self-belief. When it came to the pushing stage, one woman,

Sabine, I spoke to, drew a comparison with surfing, where she struggled to dive underneath a wave with her board ('duck diving') and started to get agitated. She used this agitation as an extra strength to dive under the water and she explained that when she was in the pushing stage of labour, she drew on this experience to push the baby out as she had the belief that she had it in her to find the energy needed even though she was tired.

In addition to previous performance accomplishments, there are other sources that can help with your self-belief. Having role models who are in a similar situation to you and who have successfully managed the labour experience can be a very powerful source to inform your self-belief. What is important here is that the role model has been in a similar situation; otherwise, it won't help to improve your self-belief. This is quite important not only in a time where many of us have social media accounts and follow others on social media but also when attending mum-to-be groups and antenatal yoga classes. Pregnant women come in all shapes and sizes and have different stories. For example, you may have had an emergency caesarean for your first child and want to give birth vaginally for your second child, you can feel more confident when learning from other women who have gone through a similar experience. Therefore, try to find role models with a similar story to you and learn from them to help inform your self-belief.

Another source that can influence your self-efficacy is verbal persuasion; this is the impact of 'words' or encouragement and motivation through 'talk'. This can be feedback from your birth partner, midwife, doula, but it can also come from you, what you say to yourself. When I spoke to one of my Dutch friends, Imke, she explained how she combined previous experiences and verbal persuasion in the pushing stage. Thinking back about how (physically) tough the pushing stage felt, she recalled how she focused on the physical effort needed and compared it to lifting weights. During the pushing stage Imke told herself, 'I can do this, I have pushed (physical) boundaries before', which helped with her self-belief that she could keep going. Physiological arousal (and perceived effort), is another source of self-efficacy and this has to do with how strong you feel, as well as feelings of pain, fatigue, and arousal. If you have extensive experience of doing sport and exercise, you are aware how you can use breathing to manage physiological arousal and calm your body down. This knowledge of your body is very helpful. What is important to consider is that the interpretation of these sensations is what informs self-efficacy, which is also the case for emotional arousal. If you expect pain, then it does not have to influence your self-efficacy, but if the pain is much more intense than anticipated, it can impact self-efficacy in an adverse way. Chrissie Wellington (triathlete and world Ironman champion) felt that expecting that there would be pain and/or discomfort, made it easier for her to handle it, and she believed that going into the labour that she was capable of enduring the pain and discomfort. You can draw on imaginal experiences to help you feel more confident about this too.

Now I have covered the different sources of self-efficacy, I encourage you to take some time and write down what you feel informs your self-belief in relation to giving birth.

1. What do you feel are important aspects in relation to giving birth? You can think about experiencing pain, letting go, staying calm, focus on the controllables, making decisions under pressure and so on.
2. Considering these aspects, such as experiencing pain, how confident do you feel in your abilities to managing high-intensity pain?
3. What are previous experiences that you can draw on to help inform your self-belief for these?

A psychological strategy like self-talk can be very helpful to inform one's self-efficacy, especially through the source of verbal persuasion. Other strategies that can be useful are imagery, goal-setting, and breathing. These strategies will be covered in later chapters, and you can refer back to your sources of self-efficacy and pick ones that you feel you could strengthen with the help of these strategies. Remember that with all strategies, it is important that you keep practicing these in the lead-up to giving birth.

Approach orientation

So far, I have outlined that having self-belief and feeling that you have control over the situation (this is different from being in control!) are key elements of a challenge state. In addition to these two components, there is a third one, something we call 'approach orientation'. Thus, rather than sticking your head in the sand and trying to avoid the situation, an approach orientation is, very simply said, about tackling the situation head-on. Although this is a bit overly simplistic, it is about the idea that rather than having the motivation that you don't want to do something wrong ('I don't want to miss this shot'), it is about what you do want to do ('I'm going to hit the next shot in the top left corner'). Here is an example, when giving birth a lot of stuff happens that you may feel uncomfortable about, and you'd rather avoid happening. It can be that you don't want to swear or that you don't want to poo because you may feel embarrassed about this. I can tell you that this is normal and giving birth can be quite a primal experience! Rather than trying to focus on all these 'what not to do', it is much more useful to focus on what you can do, such as focusing on your breathing or allowing yourself to take the time to make a decision as opposed to ignoring having to make a decision. So, to give you another example: an avoidance orientation in relation to breathing could be that you think, 'I don't want to lose control of my breathing', whereas an approach orientation is 'during the contraction I will take 5 breaths where I breath in for 6 and breath out for 6 seconds'. The key difference here is that you focus on what you are going to do and not feel anxious about something that you are trying so hard to avoid. Sometimes avoiding can feel as the easiest solution, yet focusing a lot on what you do not want to do can take a lot of energy! Think about a tennis player who is trying not to hit the ball in the net, and is so focused on that, that he or she ends up hitting the ball in the net. What's more useful, is to focus on where you want to place the ball on the opposite end of the court!

Okay, now we know that perceived control, self-belief, and an approach orientation are useful when it comes to a positive challenge. So what? Well, when it comes to challenge and threat states, we know that a challenge state (in a sport setting) is generally more helpful than a threat state; this is reflected not only by our emotional states but also by our physiological states. In a challenge state, you generally feel more positive emotions and perceive negative emotions to be more helpful. That is, you can feel anxious but also understand that it may have a purpose and that it can be beneficial. Yes, this can be tricky! Especially in labour it can be quite common to feel anxiety. To understand that this means that you care about what happens can be a way of approaching the anxiety in a more helpful way. If you constantly worry about what may go wrong, then the anxiety is probably less helpful! We will come back to emotions, and anxiety in particular, in the next chapter.

From our research, we also know that a challenge state has a more beneficial physiological component to it compared to a threat state. When it comes to labour, you don't want to have your body work harder than it already does, and therefore it can be helpful to try to work towards a challenge state. In addition, oxytocin is generally considered to be helpful in labour. It is actually nicknamed the love drug! This is helpful to know as a challenge state is suggested to be linked to more oxytocin.

What I will do in the subsequent chapters is to share some of the psychological strategies that we have used in sport psychology settings to help athletes approach situations as a challenge, or move from a threat to a challenge. I also share strategies I have used when working with endurance athletes; this can be relevant considering the comparison of giving birth to marathons!

Take-home message

1. The maternity journey can bring about a lot of physical and mental demands. Rather than seeing these demands as a threat, you can draw on self-belief, perceived control, and approach motivation as useful ingredients to create more of a challenge state. This can be helpful because a challenge state can benefit physiological responses.

2. In the lead-up to giving birth, spend some time to reflect on how you can build your self-belief. Can you do something like breathing practice to give you the confidence to breathe through pain and discomfort? What are other things that you can do to realise what you do and don't have control over?

3. Throughout the rest of the book, we cover a range of psychological strategies. You can consider which psychological strategies would help you to move to a challenge state.

3 Checking in with your emotions

If you have given birth before or spoken to women who have gone through the experience, you may have heard stories that compare the experience with an emotional rollercoaster. How can you learn to navigate this emotional rollercoaster? Imagine the excitement when the first contractions are starting, happiness about meeting the baby soon, perhaps anxiety about what is to come, frustration or even anger when things are not going as planned, and the elation, joy, or relief when the baby is born. When I think about my experience, I can feel my heart rate increase when I think back about the moment that I was told I was going to be transported to the labour room to be induced without having had a conversation with anyone about what was to come yet. It made me angry at the time as I felt so out of control and wanted to understand what was happening. I also recall feeling a bit annoyed with myself when I lost focus when trying to tune in to the pain during a contraction, followed by feeling rather pleased when I was able to refocus. Goosebumps still appear when I recall the moment that I pushed my baby out, my emotions were all over the place, but a combination of elation, surprise and pride probably describes it best.

Emotional rollercoasters are also common in sports. Let's take running a marathon – there is the anxiety before the start to the elation when crossing the finish line, and then all the emotions in between. This could be the excitement and racing off a little too fast at the start of the race, denial after throwing your pacing or nutrition plan out of the window, maybe some anger when a 'helpful' supporter tells a runner that there is 'only' half of the marathon left to go, to the desperation when a runner hits the wall, perhaps wanting to give up, and then finding the power to keep going. Of course, a big difference with a marathon is that giving up is not quite that easy when you are in labour and about to push a baby out or if you are getting ready to have a C-section. You also don't always know exactly how long it will be until the finish line or how many detours you may have to take. Although a lot of the research on emotions in relation to pregnancy and giving birth has focused on the fluctuating emotions during pregnancy and the time after giving birth, post-partum, the emotions experienced during childbirth are important to consider as these emotions can have an impact on how you look back at the experience. In this chapter, we will have a look at how emotions work and what some approaches are to managing emotions.

The emotional rollercoaster – what are emotions about?

Why can labour be such an emotional rollercoaster? Let's start with a short overview of how emotions work. First, it is important to acknowledge that emotions are very complex! As a very basic explanation, emotions are a reaction to an event that triggers us, this 'stimulus' or trigger event can be real or something we imagine. It involves changes in our body, such as increased heart rate, breathing rate, sweating, and everyone experiences emotions in their own way. You often notice that emotions are expressed through facial changes and actions, perhaps a change in body posture, tensing up or moving your face away if you feel upset. An emotion is a response to a trigger event. For example, you may have performed really well in a competition and felt happy about this. Maybe you think about what it would be like to meet your baby for the first time, and you feel excited about this. Perhaps you have lost a baby during a previous pregnancy and the thought of this makes you feel very upset and scared. This is understandable and it is okay to feel upset about this situation. Or you might think about the potential of giving birth in the car because when you were born, it all happened super quickly, and the thought of having your baby in a car makes you feel very anxious. What this shows is that emotions can be, but are not always, linked to something that has happened or is currently ongoing; and emotions can relate to your thoughts.

In line with this idea that emotions are a response to an event, or a response to something that has happened, one way through which you can understand the process around emotions is by what is called 'primary and secondary appraisals'. The quote by Shakespeare in Hamlet, 'Nothing is either good or bad, but thinking makes it so' illustrates appraisals quite well. Appraisals are like judgements and consist of two main aspects; an evaluation of the *event* (like a stressor) and an evaluation of the *coping options* available to you. Together, these evaluations influence how you feel about the situation, and as such appraisals are a bit like the story behind your emotions. I will break this down a bit more for you, as it can be helpful to reflect on both what's at stake and what you perceive to have available to manage the situation.

First, primary appraisals have to do with your evaluation of an event; this evaluation is what influences how you feel about the situation. Primary appraisals involve a judgement or evaluation of what is at stake, usually in relation to your well-being, and these evaluations help you to identify the relevance of the situation. If giving birth at home is important to you, but your contractions start well before your due date when you are out and about, and you have to go to the hospital instead, you could see this as a potential for growth (you will be in good care, will be looked after, and can fully focus on the strategies that you have practiced to birth your baby) or a potential for harm (you have not packed your hospital bag and feel uncomfortable in a different setting). In essence, what happens at this stage is a decision on whether you evaluate what's going on as something that is important to you, and if so, whether the situation presents a threat, with potential for harm, or potential for gain, like a positive challenge. Whether you then experience negative emotions like worry and anxiety or positive emotions like excitement depends on the secondary appraisal.

Secondary appraisals are about evaluating the options available to you to deal with the event or situation and a consideration of how effective these options would be. If you do not feel that you have the coping resources to deal with the situation or you think that these coping resources would not work in this situation, then you are more likely to experience negative emotions such as anxiety and frustration. On the other hand, if you feel that you can do something that helps to prevent harm or threat, and could lead to benefits or a positive challenge, then this could lead to experiencing positive emotions, such as happiness or excitement. In essence, this is what coping is about, making efforts to reduce or get rid of this possible harm.

All of this may feel a bit abstract. To help give you an idea of primary and secondary appraisals, below you will find some questions that you can use to reflect on situations that may trigger strong emotional reactions. The reflection can help to give you an insight into what it is about the situation that leads to triggering a strong emotional reaction, and to think about the coping options available to you. To give you an idea of how it works, I have used a personal example that I come back to later in the chapter as well.

Primary appraisals	Explanation
Is there something at stake? If so, what is it? Is this important to me? What is the potential impact on me?	What is the situation? Why does it matter to me? Is the situation impacting my well-being? How does the situation affect me? Does the situation compromise my values or the goals I have? Is the situation harmful, or can I get some benefits out of the situation?
	Example: My water has broken, there is no sign of regular contractions, which means that I will need to be induced and I won't be able to get the 'no-intervention' birth experience that I had hoped for. This compromises my goal of being active during birth and I may be missing out on an intimate birth experience. There is potential for harm considering that there are some risks to the baby if the water is broken, especially if the baby poos in the womb, and it feels like there is no opportunity for shared decision-making with the medical staff, taking away my autonomy and desire for a collaborative experience.

(Continued)

(Continued)

Secondary appraisals	Explanation
What are your existing coping resources? Can I control the situation? What are my future expectations?	Do I have potential to cope with the situation? What do I have available to me and what do I expect will come out of these coping options? If I do X, will that make the situation better? What is controllable, what is not controllable? If you have identified a potential for harm or a threat, is this something that you can remove? Is there scope to move from a threat to a challenge?

Example: Yes, I do have potential to cope with the situation and I am aware that what the baby does is outside of my control, but I also realise that I have options available to me and I can still take ownership over how I manage parts of the situation. I know that my partner will be there for me no matter what and that he will support me in my decision-making. I know I have the right to ask for some time with my partner to make decisions. I will also give myself some time and space to feel upset about the birth experience that I was aiming for, but I should not fight being induced as I know that getting myself in fight or flight mode will make the situation worse. Having a good cry and then telling myself 'it will be a different birth and that's okay', will help me to refocus and find ways I can still make the most out of the experience, such as giving it my best effort to give birth with as little pain relief as I can reasonably manage. |
| Conclusion | Okay, so I won't get the birth experience that I was hoping for, I know that the water has broken and things need to get moving. What the baby does is outside of my control, and at the end of the day I want to give birth to a healthy baby. I can draw on a range of coping options that I know will help me – I have a supportive partner, I can stand up for myself, so I still feel I have autonomy, and I can still try to give birth without too much pain relief so I can feel the baby's head coming out. So actually, I can turn this into a positive challenge. |

The emotional rollercoaster – anxiety

So now I have given you some background about emotions, let's have another ride on the rollercoaster of emotions. On this rollercoaster, one of the emotions that women often refer to is anxiety. Anxiety is an emotion that is associated with worry, apprehension, and tension in the body. Although anxiety gets a lot of bad press, experiencing a little bit of anxiety can serve a protective function. Sometimes anxiety can be like a warning signal and may lead to holding back, which is not always a bad thing. You can think about it as having an 'anxiety sweet spot', where some anxiety is okay, but too much anxiety can become problematic. Anxiety can also be an indication that you care, and you can decide to interpret it as such. Anxiety is one of the most researched topics in sport psychology. Broadly, a distinction is made between two types of anxiety: *cognitive*, which has to do with thoughts such as worries, and *somatic* anxiety, which has to do with physical and physiological symptoms, such as feeling tension in the body or an increased heart rate. Interestingly, research consistently finds that when sportspeople are asked to report their anxiety levels when thinking about an upcoming competition that this cognitive anxiety can be experienced well before the actual competition. Somatic anxiety, however, is often not experienced intensely until the competition comes closer and becomes more intense and often peaks an hour or so before the competition starts. Knowing that cognitive and somatic anxiety may peak at different times is useful, so that you can reflect on what your 'anxiety sweet spot' is for cognitive and somatic anxiety in potentially stressful situations. Knowing about this is helpful as you can adapt the strategies used to manage anxiety, for example, breathing exercises (chapter 7) could help with too much somatic anxiety close to the start or during a stressful situation, and using self-talk (chapter 6) or acceptance (chapter 7) can be a good strategy for managing cognitive anxiety. Distraction strategies (chapter 8) in the week before may be useful to take your mind away from cognitive anxiety if it starts to get a bit much. Do note, however, that if anxiety consistently takes over and you can't draw on any strategies to manage your anxiety levels, then you need to take action. This is not a medical book – when anxiety interferes with your day-to-day life, it is really important to discuss this with a health professional and let people in your environment know.

What triggers your anxiety? As you learnt at the start of this chapter, emotions are a reaction to a 'trigger event', and anxiety is no different. To help manage anxiety, it is helpful to reflect on where the anxiety might come from. Having an awareness of this will help to work on the source of the anxiety rather than just trying really hard to suppress the emotion (anxiety or another emotion that you might feel is unhelpful). If you try to suppress or push away the emotion, then it may be gone temporarily. There may be times that pushing your emotions aside can be useful, even necessary, but in the long term this will cost a lot of effort. Suppressing emotions could also result in the emotion coming back at an inconvenient time or even returning more forcefully. A common analogy for this is that of trying to push a beachball under the water. You can keep pushing, but eventually that beachball will pop out of the water again, and often with quite some force. Some of the things that might influence anxiety in the context of childbirth are how you experience pain, feelings of having to let go of control, and thinking about what can go wrong during the birth. This is no surprise, because we sometimes seem to hear and tune in to negative birth stories more so than positive birth stories, and the negative birth stories often have a bigger impact, and as such, these tend to stick with us. From an evolutionary perspective, this is quite normal; we tend to focus on (perceived) threats. There are, however, plenty of positive birth stories, and we need to start focusing more on these rather than waiting for those negative stories. That is, you can take a proactive role and search for positive birth stories to make you feel more empowered.

If we start with pain as a factor that can fuel anxiety, what is important to be aware of is that there are big differences in how women experience pain during labour. In chapter 1, I explained that the concept of pain has several components, such as pain *tolerance* (amount of pain you are able to tolerate until it becomes too much), pain *threshold* (minimum point that you perceive something as being painful), and pain *intensity* (magnitude of pain). These three components play a role in how you experience pain, and it is a very personal thing. For some women, it is like nothing they have ever experienced before, despite having conquered pain and discomfort in and outside of their sport. Especially when there is very little time in between contractions, and it feels like it is a 'storm' of contractions with no break in between, it can be quite intense. This feeling of being overwhelmed by pain can fuel anxiety if you are unsure how to handle the pain or if you feel misunderstood by the people around you. What is also very relevant in this context is that, when you are feeling overwhelmed by pain, it can be very difficult to verbally communicate your levels of pain and get the right support for you. This can then fuel anxiety further. One woman I spoke with, Alda, explained how she felt anxious and very tense when she was giving birth to her first child. From previous conversations with her mum, she was getting worried that she might give birth very quickly and much quicker than the average person because of her family history. As the contractions got intense rather quickly, there was no time to gradually adapt to the pain. She also felt that she was working against her body, by rolling into a ball like a hedgehog and clenching her muscles, which could have easily made the pain more intense. With her second child, she was aware that the anxiety was working against the pain, she was taking action in letting the medical staff know about how quickly her labour could progress just in case, and in the lead-up to getting her epidural, she was telling herself that yes it's painful, but let the body do the work and get through the wave.

A few other women I spoke to compared the labour pain to (sport) injury pain and felt that this experience prepared them to adapt and manage the pain. They realised that pain was part of the process and did not feel threatened by it. As such, they felt they could draw on some of those experiences when they suffered from pain and knew that they would be able to see this through and used acceptance as a way to manage the pain. Chrissie Wellington (ironman triathlete) explained how the power of recollection helped her to manage the pain and discomfort; she knew she had overcome pain and discomfort in training and in previous races. Knowing in the birthing process what she had endured as an athlete was very empowering. She knew that she had done this before, which gave her piece of mind and the comfort that she could endure it again. She also knew that she had an uncomplicated labour so far and had complete trust in her support team. This is another example of how these primary and secondary appraisals I talked about earlier work together – she evaluated that there was no harm, the baby was doing well, and she felt she could manage the controllables in the situation, as such she felt more positive and helpful emotions. Similarly, Amy Williams (skeleton Olympic gold medallist) reflected on how much pain she had to endure in her sport, from bad delayed onset of muscle soreness to her knee injury, which she described as some of the worst pain in her life. This helped her to view the pain as something that would stop, it would not last forever, and she reminded herself that the contractions and pain were part of the process to help deliver her baby. Drawing on her knowledge of the physiological and psychological processes that happen during labour, Pip (midwife and runner) explained that this helped her to accept the (physiological) processes; she would see the contractions as a powerful part, rather than a painful process, and she did not perceive them as a threat. She also explained that this acceptance was beneficial for keeping up endorphins, which is a useful hormone when it comes to pain relief.

During pregnancy and childbirth, there is a lot of uncertainty, which is normal, yet it can make you feel out of control as it's difficult to plan for. Comparisons with others and feeling out of control, or having to let go of control, can be big factors that can influence our emotions. For example, other women with a similar due date have had their baby already and you become increasingly anxious about when it is your turn. Unless you have a planned intervention (like a C-section), it is quite different from sports where you often have a set date that you can prepare for. Funmi (personal trainer) illustrated how comparisons to others could fuel unhelpful emotions. When she was on the ward after being induced and waiting for things to happen, she saw other women who arrived on the ward after her going into the labour room before her, and she thought 'why is this woman going to have her baby before me, it should be my turn by now'. This can make you feel anxious or even frustrated, when you are comparing yourself to others, and it may not go as you'd like. This is also linked to control, and it can suppress the release of endorphins. Control can play such a big role in the birth process, all this uncertainty and feeling out of control can be hard and make you feel anxious. Especially when you feel that you are in the hands of health professionals, this can make you feel vulnerable especially if you are in an unfamiliar environment. But what is important is that you can consider this beforehand and plan for the emotional rollercoaster. Having an awareness of what the types of things are that you can control and plan for, and what those uncontrollable things are, can help with easing some of this anxiety as you don't try to, unsuccessfully, control the uncontrollables. If you know that letting go of control is a big thing fuelling your anxiety and confidence, then it is important to think about how you can manage that.

It is important to note that despite this rollercoaster of emotions, there is a lot of scope for more research on how to ride this rollercoaster. As research often drives informational resources that are available, what does this mean? Firstly, having more resources available on this can help normalise your feelings, it is okay to experience emotions, and there are ways to manage these. Secondly, the people around you, such as the medical team, your partner, or family may not be in tune with your emotions. That is not completely unexpected as the medical team is typically trained and focused on the physiological aspects of birth and makes their decisions accordingly. Your partner and family may be dealing with their own feelings and emotions and as such find it hard to tune in to your emotions. Having said that, it is helpful if those around you are catering to your emotional needs as the emotional rollercoaster does not always align with the physiological rollercoaster of giving birth. Although I come back to perceived social support later in this book, I wanted to raise it here already. Most (birth)partners do want to be there for you and want to give you that emotional support, but let's not forget that it can be a very emotional experience for them too. Therefore, you might find it helpful to have a chat with whoever will be present when you give birth and share how both of you think you will respond emotionally in different scenarios.

So perhaps you have started to think about how emotions can influence what you do, maybe when you feel anxious you act a bit flustered, or you might find it difficult to think clearly and make decisions. Maybe you feel your heart rate increases, or perhaps when you are angry you feel that your body tenses up. You may have experienced this when playing sports, your reaction time got a bit too fast when overly excited or you fumbled a ball because you felt angry after a poor call by the umpire. But did you know that there is a lot more going on in your body when you have these emotions? Although this is not a medical book, it is important to draw your attention to the link between emotions and hormonal changes, and how this can affect the labour process. Facing a stressful situation, which can lead to emotions such as anxiety and fear, is often linked to what is called 'fight or flight'. The fight or flight is about preparing the body for this stressful or dangerous situation, where you feel your heart beats faster, you get sweaty hands, and so on. Although this fight or flight response helps to prepare your body for action, what this can do is stall 'optimal conditions' for progressing the labour. I remember that when I had more regular contractions, we jumped into a taxi and went back to the hospital in the early hours of the morning. After an initial wait, they monitored the baby and my contractions for 30 minutes and my contractions just completely stalled. I was getting worried that my plan of having a calm birth in the birth centre was not going to happen, and to be honest, I think at this stage, I was trying to control an uncontrollable situation as my water had already broken some time ago, and I starting to get into fight or flight mode. Not the most helpful state! The midwife in the birth centre told us to go back home again rather than waiting it out in the hospital as the home environment would be calm and more relaxed, so back we went. She encouraged me to try to see if I could express some colostrum and explore other ways to increase my oxytocin, which is needed during the labour process and to get contractions going. In fact, when you are being induced with a 'hormone drip', this is what you will be getting, an artificial form of oxytocin called syntocinon. As we were given a 'deadline' of when to come back to the hospital, there was not really space for feeling relaxed, and despite trying to make the bedroom dark and watching a romcom, I felt anything but relaxed, nor do I think that my oxytocin levels were particularly high!

What was important here is that I was, after a while, able to let go. I was very upset that I could not give birth in the birth centre. I then allowed myself some space to feel upset before we set off in the taxi again (for the third time) to go to the labour ward. Making space for my emotions was what I needed to help manage my feelings and let go. When we were admitted to the labour ward, I was in good spirits, had a lot more clarity in my mind, I was less driven by unhelpful emotions, and I felt more confident about what was to come. It is not about controlling and suppressing your emotions, which costs a lot of energy, but about acknowledging and tuning in to your emotions. It can feel like a big step, from controlling your emotions and overthinking to tuning in to your feelings. Therefore, it is helpful to practice this in the lead-up to labour so that you feel more comfortable doing this. This is not just helpful practice for you, but also for your (birth) partner.

When it comes to emotions, there are many approaches that you can take to manage or deal with emotions. A popular approach to deal with the situation that has led to the emotion that you are experiencing is problem-focused and emotion-focused coping. I mentioned coping when I explained 'secondary appraisals', and as a simple definition, coping can be about your effort to minimise or get rid of the potential harm or threat of a situation. Now, you can do this by trying to change something about the situation and take control of it, which is what problem-focused coping is about, or you can try to manage the emotions that come with the situation, rather than trying to change the situation itself, which is emotion-focused coping. This is quite a helpful distinction to make, as you cannot always change the situation itself, and if you are trying hard to engage in problem-solving or removing the source of the stress, it can quickly turn into a bit of a downward spiral. For example, the umbilical cord may be wrapped around the baby's neck, called a nuchal chord. From my understanding of the research, this is not something you can actively prevent from happening. Engaging in active problem-solving to change the situation could therefore cost a lot of energy. It may be more helpful to move to emotion-focused coping to help stay calm and focus on the delivery. In addition, information provision, such as knowing that it happens regularly and that it is something that medical staff are experienced in dealing with, can be a helpful coping strategy for some people.

Later in the book, I cover various coping strategies – some can be used both as emotion-focused and problem-focused coping. For example, imagery can be used to imagine a happy place to calm your anxiety (emotion-focused) or to imagine the different options available to you in a situation (problem-focused coping). Thus, rather than providing you with a distinct overview of what a problem-focused coping strategy is and what an emotion-focused coping strategy is, I mostly want to emphasise for you to reflect on the coping option and whether that is helpful for you in that situation. The key message here is that not all coping strategies work all the time. This is relevant because we often tend to prefer a particular coping strategy. This can be really helpful as it is a strategy that you have practiced before and so you know how it works. Overreliance on a preferred coping strategy does have a downside though, as the same coping strategy may not work in every single situation. As such, being flexible in your coping is advocated, especially in situations where your preferred coping strategy is not appropriate. For example, your preferred coping strategy is to engage in problem-solving and to take control of a situation. In the example above, where the umbilical cord is wrapped around the baby's head, there is perhaps not much scope for problem-solving, and the control may need to be handed to the medical team to help make a decision on what is best for the baby's and the mother's health. It can be quite frustrating when you feel that your preferred coping strategy is being thwarted or undermined, but sometimes this will happen especially when there is a tricky medical situation. Therefore, I would recommend that you reflect on your preferred coping strategies and identify when these are helpful and when these are less helpful. Discuss this with important people around you, so that they can remind you of these when the 'pressure' is on. When you are calm and composed and thinking about your ideal birth, it all seems fine, but when suddenly the contractions start and come quicker than expected, it may well be that you are not as calm as you had anticipated. At the same time, you may also want to do the coping reflection tasks in this chapter with your partner, as they may be the ones who find it difficult to stay calm under pressure! You could also consider whether there are some shared coping options available to you and your (birth)partner too.

What can you do? How can you put this in practice? To summarise the key points of this chapter, I have outlined a few take-home messages that you can consider to help you be aware of your emotions, what fuels your emotions, and how you can prepare and manage your emotions.

Take-home message

1. Spend some time noticing the emotions that you are experiencing in different situations. Being aware of the variety of emotions you can experience can be a very useful step because it can help you understand why you feel happy, or perhaps feel tense and find it difficult to focus on a task or take in information.

2. Consider what it is about the situation that makes you experience this (or these) emotion(s). Here you can go back to the questions I outlined earlier in relation to understanding what's behind the emotion. Is there a potential for harm, is there a threat? What is the potential for an opportunity, or a positive challenge?

3. When trying to manage an emotion, reflect on whether there is any use in trying to change the situation. Sometimes this is a possibility, for example, you planned a home birth, but it makes you feel anxious and you decide to change the delivery mode and

go to the birth centre in a hospital. Sometimes there is very little that you can change about the situation; think about a situation where the baby is in a position that requires an intervention that you had not anticipated, and an emotion-focused coping strategy may be more effective.

4. Think about what coping strategies are already available to you, or are there any other strategies you could adopt? In the upcoming chapters, you can learn more about goal-setting, imagery, self-talk, relaxation and breathing, mindfulness-based techniques, and attention control, and reflect on whether these are strategies that you could use.

5. Reflect on whether there are certain types of coping that you typically fall back on. If so, think about whether there are events during labour when these coping strategies are perhaps less useful, so that you can put together a backup plan with strategies that you could use if your 'standard' coping option does not work.

4 Birth plan overboard! Goal-setting and goal-revision

How do you want to give birth? Where do you want to give birth? Do you want a water birth? When is your caesarean section? Who do you want with you during your labour? What birthing equipment are you intending to use? Do you want to have immediate skin-to-skin contact with your baby? What pain relief do you want? When you are putting together a birth plan, these are just some of the questions to consider. Planning for labour is a big part of the preparation, and you may set yourself goals for how you want to approach the birth of your child.

Goal-setting is one of the most popular strategies in sport and performance psychology. In a nutshell, goal-setting is about figuring out what it is that you want to achieve and to identify a plan on how you will get there. When we think about goal-setting, the focus often ends up being on the outcome and much less on how to get there. What this focus on the outcome leads to is that the journey ends up being forgotten about. The reason I believe that this can be unfortunate is that it is draining energy (dare I say motivation) if you can't see light at the end of the tunnel or constantly feel you are lost, but let's also remember that the roads on the way to a destination are an important part of your journey. I am not going to say that the road is always pretty, but there can be many precious moments along the way if we make an effort to tune in to the journey and not just the outcome. In this chapter, I will share some different ways you can use goal-setting and how you can work on mapping out your route. Before I share the different ways of applying goal-setting, I will focus on the 'quality' of goals, because I believe that it is as much about the quality of the goal and the meaningfulness of the goals as it is about how you map out your journey.

Quality of goals

Just having 'a goal' is not sufficient for goals to work properly. A goal needs to be meaningful to you and serve a relevant purpose. Some goals are intended to give you that initial boost to get started, whereas other goals are more specific, like how you want to manage pain. As such, there are different types of goals and these serve different purposes. In sports, a common differentiation is made between goals that focus on outcomes, such as finishing position or your time, and process goals. Outcome goals that have to do with finishing position, such as winning the league or a race or beating someone, can give that initial energy boost to your motivation, but it is a goal that you do not have a big amount of control over, as you are dependent on others in the league or race. If beating others is important to you, then this is probably a goal that you are familiar with. It can be a great feeling when you do beat others, but it can lead to feeling dissatisfied and other negative emotions such as frustration and anxiety that can impact your well-being when you don't win or succeed. Although you may not see a direct link between this type of goal and giving birth, you'd be surprised. For some people, comparisons to others are really important as to how they define success and perceive that they are doing well. For example, they may set themselves a goal to give birth in a 'better way' than someone else (this could be a sibling, or whoever!), give birth before someone else in their antenatal class with a similar due date (not particularly controllable!), or be back exercising more quickly than someone else. This is not within your control, and arguably not that helpful.

In sports, it is also common to set goals that focus on performance compared to your own standards, such as running a 10 km under 55 minutes. This type of goal is something you can have more control over. Having said that, if your performance goal is to be fully dilated in a certain time frame, then perhaps less so. Hence it is important to set realistic goals, and we will get to that later. Finally, process goals are about *how* you are getting to your destination. Thus, you may set a performance goal of giving birth, considering baby and mother are happy and healthy, with as little intervention as feasible, and the route to this, the *how* is to remind yourself of your breathing strategy at regular intervals. Process goals are an important one, as it will give you a lot more control over the situation. You want to set process goals that are manageable. For example, wanting to stay calmer than before, you can set a process goal to count to six whilst taking a deep breath when you feel that you are losing your calm, or you can set a process goal of moving to a different labour position when you are transitioning to the pushing stage of labour. So, really when we consider setting goals, I would advocate that you focus on process goals and ditch any goals where you compare yourself to others or those other goals that are very much outside of your control. There are so many more important things than comparing yourself to others, and although I draw comparisons with sport in this book, let's remember that giving birth is NOT a competition!

What to consider when setting goals?

Goal-setting is a strategy, and this is one that you can learn. Rather than moving straight to setting a goal, when you start thinking about goals, there are a few aspects to consider, such as making sure that the goals are realistic and adaptable, within your perceived control, specific, and meaningful to you. I'd also like to add that wherever feasible, try to make goals enjoyable! What is important when setting a realistic goal is that you base the goal on what you are capable of (remember self-efficacy) and take into consideration your recent circumstances. This is so easy to overlook, but so important! Babies keep moving and wiggling around, so their positioning may change and this could, for example, influence the goal you may have set of having a particular type of birth. Or perhaps you planned for a caesarean section delivery, but the last couple of weeks have been going well and you now feel like trying to go for a vaginal birth, or the baby decides to want to come out earlier than the planned date for the C-section. All of that can happen! Therefore, it is important that goals are set in a way that these can be adapted. Ensure that there is 'wiggle' room for goals, so that rather than throwing a birth plan completely overboard, you can adapt it and you feel that you can control some of the controllables.

Another way of looking at setting adaptable goals is explained by Amy Williams, illustrating this both in a birthing as well as a skeleton context:

> *You have got your best scenario, now make up the second scenario, like A, B, and C. The perfect birth, the not quite so perfect, and what could be the worst example. So at least you have gone through them in your head, you are prepared, you visualise each of these experiences. So if plan A does not happen, okay I can accept that and move straight onto plan B and I have already accepted plan B in my head because I have already rehearsed it. That is what I did on the track, I'd enter a corner on the skeleton track either in my perfect position or crap I am a bit too left, so what am I going to do now to change my steers? Okay, I have not come out very well so what am I now going to do to change as fast as possible.*

In my work with endurance runners, I often compare this to levels of goals, where you might set a dream (gold) goal, a happy (silver) goal, and an okay (bronze) goal. A dream goal is when all the conditions are ideal, such as good weather, feeling well-rested, adequate nutrition, and plenty of positive energy. But sometimes, not everything goes as expected, perhaps you get carried away at the start or it is a very humid and hot day and you revert to your happy goal. Or maybe if it feels like a less-than-ideal day, you have slept poorly, food does not sit well in your stomach, and your legs feel heavy, you may then decide to move to the okay goal. Having prepared for it can make it easier to keep going and don't let unfavourable circumstances get to you that much. You can of course also move up from an okay goal to a happy or dream goal.

You can consider engaging your midwife, doula, obstetrician, gynaecologist, and others with expertise around you when you are setting your goals to help understand what makes a realistic goal. You can think about how these people can help you to set realistic goals, especially as they have a wealth of knowledge to provide insights into at what stage of labour goals are most likely to be adapted when giving birth. Seeing the midwife as a collaborative partner in this process can give you confidence, and writing down the goals in your maternity notes will serve as a reminder to you and the team around. This may be more difficult to do when you see a different midwife at every appointment, as is the case in some places, yet you could write down your goals and discuss these at your antenatal appointments.

When setting a goal, it is also important to think about who has set the goal or influenced you to set this goal. In an ideal world, you want to set goals that are aligned with what's important to you, such as your values, and set goals that 'belong' to you. In essence, these are goals that you perceive to be within your control. You could label these as *autonomous* goals. On the other hand, there are 'controlled goals', these are goals that are set for you by others and that you feel controlled by. It could be that these goals are set for you by health practitioners, your midwife, your partner, your family, or it could be a societal thing. For example, in some societies, it is common to have a caesarean section; in others, to have a home birth or to have as little medicated pain intervention as possible. Let's also not underestimate how social media can 'control' your goals. You may see birth stories from other mothers, and feel the pressure that you have to give birth in a similar fashion. Social media can be a wonderful medium and provide support, but remember that it is not a comparison game, and giving birth is a very personal and individual experience. It is about *you* and you are ultimately the one who has grown this baby inside your womb.

This leads me on to the next consideration, which is about setting goals that are meaningful to you and that you are passionate about. Setting a goal that you are passionate about will make it easier to stick with this goal. I will give a personal example here. One of my labour goals was to have a vaginal birth with as little medical pain intervention for as long as possible as I wanted to experience feeling the baby coming out and reduce the chances of tearing (mind you, not all of this is *that* controllable!). Although in my birth plan I had planned a water birth in the birth centre, I was also aware that although I had a low-risk pregnancy, anything could happen in the lead-up to labour, such as the baby moving to a breech position or being in distress. However, being passionate about wanting to feel the baby come out of me was so important to me that it informed behaviours and process goals I set in the lead-up to labour, followed by decision-making when my water broke and I had to abandon my scenario A, the 'dream birth plan'. These process goals included planning breathing strategies, setting goals for exercise and sleep, knowledge gathering for how to reduce chances of tearing and so on. I then ended up with a combination of bigger and smaller mini goals that I felt helped to put me in a good position. Doing so would make it easier for me to accept if I needed to abandon my plan. I am not going to say this was easy, and I did shed a tear or two when I had to adapt my plan, but I knew that there were still things that I could do and feel empowered over to make the birthing process as meaningful to me as possible. Understanding your values are helpful to set goals that are meaningful to you. Values are principles that guide us and are about what you want to do and how you want to do it. In essence, it is about deep down in our hearts how you want to interact and connect with others around you, with yourself and with the world. To gain some clarity around your values, you can ask yourself questions such as how do you want to be in your interactions and relationships with others, what is it that you want to stand for in life, if someone really close and important to you would give a speech on one of your milestone birthdays or a big event like a wedding, what would you want them to say? Gaining clarity around your values is not necessarily easy, yet it can be a helpful exercise.

Ideally, you'd like your values and behaviour to be in harmony, that is, what you do is in line with what you want to stand for in life. You may find that sometimes your values can pull you in different directions. That does not mean that you have to change your values radically, but sometimes you want to find a compromise. There may be situations where one value may have to take precedence over another. Let me give you an example, imagine that being independent, perseverant, and safety are important values to someone. In preparation for an upcoming competition, you have planned one last intense training session. Your knee is bothering you a bit and you feel discomfort where it starts to turn into a slippery slope between good pain and bad pain, do you keep going (perseverance) and doing this by yourself (independence), or do you not want to take the risk of getting an injury (safety) and slow down, or stop, and perhaps schedule an appointment with a physiotherapist? Similarly, in labour, imagine that you are always driven by perseverance and not giving up. There is not much progress, and you have tried hard for a very long time and starting to get very tired and tense. There is a choice to keep trying or to have assistance, which may be in your best interest. What do you do, and how much will you be guided by your values?

The other recommendation I would make when setting goals, especially when it comes to process goals, is to set goals that are specific. When goals are vague and unclear, it can be difficult to commit and follow through on the goals. In sport settings, examples of specific goals can be to run a negative split in your next running session, stick to a particular pacing plan when cycling, implement an offensive play in basketball leading to a great pass for a free shot, be able to run at an 8 out of 10 in terms of perceived effort for two minutes longer than last week and so on. When it comes to labour, you may have set yourself a goal of staying positive throughout. When you think about this, it is quite a vague goal. What is it that you intend to stay positive about, and is this throughout the lead-up, during, and/or after labour? What you want to stay positive about could vary drastically depending on the situation. For example, do you want to stay positive when you are well over the due date? Then a specific goal may be to focus on what you can do to keep yourself and the baby happy and set specific process goals for this, which could be to eat healthily, monitor your body, rest, and perhaps if your body allows it, to do some gentle exercise or stretching. Jo, one of the mothers I interviewed, was more than a week over her due date, and had agreed with her medical team to push back her caesarean-section date as she was hoping that she could deliver her baby vaginally after having had her first child delivered by emergency C-section. As the C-section date came closer, she had set her mind on doing things that were fun. One of these was a choir performance at 41 weeks and 2 days pregnant, which ended up being two days before she ended up giving birth! This was a specific goal of doing an activity that would keep her positive, but at the same time, it was also a flexible goal where she did not feel the pressure to do the event if she did not feel like it.

Finally, it is helpful to consider setting both long-term and short-term goals. A long-term goal that is quite far away might feel intimidating, and this is where setting short-term goals can come in. The majority of babies are born between 37 and 41 weeks of pregnancy, and thinking about this can feel rather intimidating when you are at the start of your maternity journey. Similarly, focusing on how long the average woman is in labour can feel daunting. To help make a longer-term goal more manageable, you can do something that is called 'chunking', which is simply said breaking up the journey into smaller steps or segments with different milestones along the way. It may be that one of these is when contractions are becoming more regular, approximately three contractions every ten minutes, that you will ring the midwife. Another way you can use chunking is for when contractions are more regular, at this stage it is quite typical that a contraction lasts around a minute with a two or three-minute 'rest' before the next contraction, although this does vary from person to person. You can use chunking to break up the one-minute contractions into different parts; there is the first part of the contraction, where the intensity starts to ramp up, where you can focus on breathing or active movement (whatever works for you), up to the maximum intensity of the contraction where you might want to really put all your effort into managing the pain intensity, followed by a reduction of the intensity of the contraction. If you are in a situation where the contractions are being monitored, you can also try to use the screen to break down the contractions. For example, your birth partner can let you know when the peak of the contraction is behind you and you can start to relax again. This can be a bit tricky as not every peak is the same, clockwatching does not work for everyone, and some women barely get a rest in between contractions, so it really depends on your personal situation. Doing this could make a minute a lot more manageable, especially if you know that you will have a rest where you can maybe take a sip of water or close your eyes and rest.

Chunking is a method of goal-setting that was really useful for me at a stage of labour when I really had enough and felt that there was no end in sight. When I was induced and breathing and focusing my way through the contractions, the midwife told me, after five or six hours of contractions (and two days after the water broke) that things were progressing well and that the baby should probably be out in three hours or so. I had to let that sink in for a second. She told me that the end is in sight, but you still have a long way to go, and I also was in quite a bit of discomfort by then. As a sport psychologist who works with endurance runners, the last thing to mention to a marathon runner is that they are nearly there when they still have at least a third of the marathon ahead of them! After a deep breath (and another contraction or two where I definitely lost the will to focus on my breathing), I regrouped and my partner and I calculated that it would take around 60 contractions. This felt like a lot, but what it did is that it helped to break down the journey and to see it as small steps rather than an endless tunnel and every contraction was a step forward on the journey. I managed to refocus and stopped looking at the clock (which was almost like the 'end of the road') as that was just not helpful at all. Chrissie Wellington also highlighted how she used chunking, drawing from her experiences as an ironman athlete where she divided races into manageable portions. She would never see an ironman as an ironman, but broke it down, to go from one swim buoy to another, or for the run to break it up in four lots of 10K, or it could be the next aid station. In relation to giving birth, she said she used this experience to break down the contractions and focus on the process goal of staying in the moment, by not thinking too far ahead.

In summary, I would suggest the following considerations when it comes to setting a goal:

1. Set goals that are realistic and that you can adapt if the situation changes
2. Set goals that are within your control
3. Set goals that are meaningful to you and that you are passionate about
4. Set goals that are specific
5. Set long-term and short-term goals

Your labour goals

What are goals that you have for labour? You may have already started to think about your birth plans and included goals as part of your birth plan. If you have not thought about your birth plan yet, and want to have one, you can take some time to think about this. Once you have an idea of your birth plan, think about which goals will help you to make your birth plan as successful to you as possible. An example of a goal may be to have a supportive environment or to stay strong and calm. Once you have thought about labour goals, write down the three goals that you feel most strongly about.

Now, let's have a closer look at these goals, taking into account the goal-setting considerations that I covered earlier in the chapter.

For each goal, think about the following questions.

1. How realistic is the goal? One way you could think about this is as follows: When you think about the likelihood that you could achieve the goal, how realistic is this on a ten-point scale? If you feel it's quite far off, is there scope to get closer to 10 in the lead-up to birth? If you don't feel that this is the case, then you may want to rethink the goal.
2. How adaptable is the goal? Is there some level of flexibility or is it very much a black-or-white goal? Are you comfortable having to make some adaptations to the goal?
3. How much do you feel you have control over the goal? Is the goal something that you want and can achieve, or is the goal very much controlled by external factors or other people? If you don't

feel you have control over the goal, then a goal can end up being something that can cause pressure instead of being helpful.

4. How meaningful is the goal? To help you with this question, you can think about who have you set the goal for? How does this goal align with your values and what is important to you? Having a goal that means something to you makes it easier to pursue the goal. If you don't really care about the goal, then it is probably not going to help you that much.

5. How specific is the goal? Is it something that can help inform your behaviour? Or is the goal vague and does not really give you much context? If the goal is too vague, it is difficult to know what you need to do.

Reflecting on these questions can help you to set goals that might work better for you. If you need to adapt goals, that's fine too. Don't feel that you need to set lots and lots of goals; a few well-considered goals are often just what you need. You might find it helpful to speak with your (birth)partner and your health practitioners, such as your midwife or a good friend who has given birth before about your goals. Verbalising and writing down goals can be helpful to remind you of the goals as well.

If-then planning: A strategy to help you follow through on your goals

To help with following-through on your goals, there is a strategy called if-then planning. As part of working on goal processes with (endurance) athletes, I also use 'implementation-intentions' better known as if-then planning. It is a strategy that focuses on goal pursuit and is used a lot in the field of health psychology, for example, when managing food habits, or getting people to become and stay physically active. Many women I have spoken to mentioned how they could not remember any of the breathing exercises that they were taught during the birth preparation classes; they just completely forgot about them during labour. So, they had good intentions, but did not act on these good intentions. These conversations were partially what inspired me to write this book. The idea of goal pursuit and if-then planning takes setting goals a step beyond just 'setting the goal'. If-then plans could help to address this issue of not acting on good intentions by making new good habits stick because you have already considered a plan. What I am also trying to get across is the idea that goal-setting is not just about the outcome but also to plan for what may happen during events, especially the unexpected.

Doesn't that sound impossible, planning for the unexpected, especially if you don't know what that may be? Let me explain how if-then planning works. An if-then plan is more specific than just setting a goal; it is about identifying situations or events that might occur and already thinking about how you will deal with that situation so that you can achieve the goal that you are aiming for. Through making if-then plans, it is like you set an intention to commit to the plan, and as such this helps you to act on your good intentions and take the desired action at the 'critical moment'. Simply said, it is to reduce the gap between good intentions and action. The example I gave earlier about Amy explaining how she had a plan A, plan B, and plan C, and having visualised what these plans look like is if-then planning in action.

An if-then plan would look as follows:

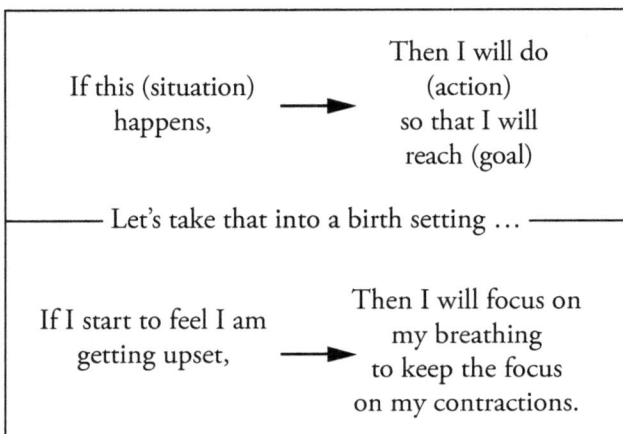

If this (situation) happens,	→	Then I will do (action) so that I will reach (goal)
— Let's take that into a birth setting ... —		
If I start to feel I am getting upset,	→	Then I will focus on my breathing to keep the focus on my contractions.

Four steps are important as part of if-then planning

1. Set a goal
2. Consider the obstacles that may get in your way (the if)
3. Come up with a plan for when this obstacle arises (the then)
4. Practice your plan

As we have already focused on setting goals, let's move on to considering the obstacles that may get in the way of your goal. Let's say that your goal is to stay calm when you are getting close to the due date but that there is a high likelihood that you may need to be induced when you are getting over your due date, which was not part of your birth plan and makes you feel anxious. What are the factors that might make it more difficult to stay calm? For example, you have heard contradicting stories about getting induced and this is worrying you. It is also quite common that people have made plans for after they have given birth based on the due date. This can vary from a trip that you have booked, family who have planned to visit for a certain date to help out, a sporting event/competition, return to work; there are so many examples of what people have planned for after labour that can impact decisions that affect your goal to stay calm. All these external factors can add a lot of pressure and can make it a lot more difficult to then accept when things do not go according to plan. The baby might find it quite comfortable in your womb and wants to stay there for a bit longer than the due date, the baby changed to a breech position just before going into labour, you may develop pregnancy diabetes and need to deliver the baby earlier than planned and so on. I do not mean to scare you and won't list all eventualities, and you may of course have a labour just as you planned, yet being aware that there is a range of factors that can get in the way, the obstacles, is helpful. Ensure that the information that you source is realistic and relevant to your personal situation. Considering which obstacles you may encounter is important because if you have not prepared for the eventuality that your labour or recovery may be different than you expected, then it can be quite tough to make changes to your birth plan in the moment.

So, that takes us to step 3, which is to come up with a plan for when the obstacle arises, and step 4, practice your plan. What is available to you to help manage the situation? Can you practice these strategies that will help you to deal with the obstacle? Practicing your plan is important, so that when you are in a situation where there may be pressure, you have access to your plan and know what to do. Some of the strategies that you could incorporate in your if-then plan will be covered later on in the book, such as self-talk, mindfulness-based techniques and imagery. I will now give you a few examples of if-then planning in action.

One woman who I spoke to whilst she was 20 weeks pregnant, Jenni (a yoga teacher and runner), explained that she was thinking about using chunking as a strategy to help with needing to adapt her running whilst pregnant. She broke down a 5K in three segments and gave herself a little reward for each completed segment. She was pondering how she could give herself rewards during labour, such as getting a head or foot massage from her partner after pushing through a set amount of contractions. In this instance, the if-then plan could look like this: 'If I struggle to find the energy to keep going then my partner will give me a head or foot massage'. Visualising that every contraction brings you one step closer to your goal of meeting the baby is another helpful way to help energise yourself and could be part of the if: 'If I struggle to find the energy to keep going, then I will visualise that with every contraction I am one step closer to meeting my baby'. I will explain imagery, sometimes known as visualisation, in chapter 5.

Another example is inspired by a pregnancy yoga teacher I had at the time who is also a doula with a wealth of knowledge. During her classes, she often emphasised how much focus there can be on how much the cervix is dilated. Of course, this could be relevant to know for the midwife, but if you are very focused on how much you are dilated, then this can turn into a big disappointment when you are not quite as far as you thought you'd be. To make a comparison with sports, you may be doing a trail run on a course that you are unfamiliar with, and you are starting to feel a bit tired and missed one of the turns. In your mind, you think that you must be close to the final couple of kilometres and you are starting to find the last bit of energy for an end spurt. Imagine the disappointment when you find out you missed your turn and you have to turn around and run further than anticipated! Maybe you just want to give up at that stage. It is not at all uncommon for that to happen. Thus, the obstacle here may be the disappointment that your cervix is not dilated by a lot. How would you then deal with this? There are a few options – one of these may be that if you know that you will be disappointed when someone tells you that you are only so far along, or that it will still take this long, then it is important to let the health practitioner know about not letting you know how many centimetres you may be dilated, as the disappoint-ment can potentially disrupt the flow and focus. Alternatively, your if-then plan could be about refocusing on your breath and accepting that you cannot force your cervix to dilate at a particular speed.

One of the things that I also encourage you to do is to prepare men-tally for the different types of births and think about how you could put this in an if-then plan. For example, if you had planned for a birth at the labour ward, but end up having a home birth because every-thing moved a little bit quicker than anticipated, it would be helpful to have planned for this eventuality beforehand. Perhaps the goal is to stay calm when contractions come on quicker than expected, and the plan (the then) would be to research the different birth options and what you can do if you were to have the baby at home. Doing so you would help you to feel less startled (although you may not have any time to feel startled if it all goes so quickly!) and gives you easier access to coping options. I would have definitely benefitted from doing more (online) tours, and to have looked at the labour ward and the opera-tion theatre in case I would have needed a C-section. When we ended up having to go the labour ward instead of the birth centre, we had initially no clue where to go! Physical tours are not always an option, especially not during a pandemic or when the times of the tours do not work for you. A silver lining of the pandemic is that, at least for a lot of hospitals here in England, virtual tours are much more available than they were before. If you do have your antenatal appointments in the hospital, you can do a recce of where the different wards are and if there are some comfortable places to go when you are waiting. If you do not have that opportunity, you could ask your midwife or someone familiar with your local birth centres or hospitals.

Take-home message

1. How can setting goals help to approach the maternity journey as a positive challenge? Here is an example, first, having gone through a few contractions and using the goal of tackling contractions one step at a time, can give you the belief that you can do it (self-belief/self-efficacy). Breaking your goal down in smaller chunks and setting the process goal of focusing on your breathing can give you a sense of perceived control. A goal like being proactive and taking each contraction one at a time can be helpful to approach, rather than avoid the situation. Together this could benefit your emotional state, where perhaps initial anxiety can turn into excitement where you can see light at the end of the tunnel and are looking forward to meeting your baby.

2. When you set goals, focus on setting good quality goals that you are passionate about. These are goals that are realistic and adaptable, within your control (control the controllables!), meaningful, and specific.

3. Setting goals is the first part of your journey, you also want to think about how you can follow-through on your goals, especially when the situation may get a bit more difficult. If-then plans can help with these situations, having already thought about how you may deal with potential obstacles makes it easier to do this when the situation arises. Ideally, you don't want to spend too much energy on figuring out how to cope with unexpected situations when you are in the middle of labour!

4. If you need to adapt your goals, that's okay. There are lots of reasons that require a (slight) change in direction, and taking a different route is not the end of the world.

5 'I could imagine the baby descending down the birth canal': Imagery as a strategy for labour and beyond

Have you ever tried to picture what it is like when the baby descends down the birth canal? Maybe you have tried to imagine what the contractions would feel like, or what the first cry of the baby sounds like. Or perhaps you have imagined yourself in a calm and peaceful place, such as a beach or the countryside, to take your mind off what's to come and to feel more relaxed. These are all examples of 'imagery', that is, the creation or recreation of an image in your mind using all your senses. You may have heard about visualisation, which is similar but relies on vision only. In this chapter, you will find out what imagery is, what ingredients of effective imagery are, and how you can use imagery.

To ensure imagery is as powerful and vivid as possible, it is important to incorporate all your senses. When I work on imagery with athletes, I focus on their awareness of the senses first. Touch, taste, sound, vision, smell, all of these senses together help to create or recreate an image in your mind. Perhaps you can imagine the squeezing of your fists (touch), the music you have chosen in the background (sound), the smell of essential oils you picked or a sweaty top (smell), a dry mouth (taste) or the cervix opening up to the size of a doughnut (vision).

Imagery can be a very powerful tool, and we use it all the time. Just think about all the times when you are walking, driving, or cycling somewhere how you imagine the route in your mind. Although we may use

Reflecting on these questions, was there one aspect that you rated yourself higher on than others? Keep that in mind as much as the aspects where you may not have rated yourself as high, as it is also important to keep building on your strengths when developing your imagery skills. Maybe you have a big dislike of lemons and so you were very aware of your feelings, or perhaps you found it difficult to generate the image to start off with, which made you feel frustrated. Reflecting on these will help you to get better at imagery in the long term.

We will come back to the basics of developing imagery later in this chapter. Before we do so, let's have a look at what you can use imagery for. Spend a couple of minutes thinking about a time when you used imagery when playing your sport. What was the purpose or reason that you used imagery? Maybe you used imagery to re-create a scenario where you felt highly energised and you used this to go into a competition with high levels of energy and positivity. Perhaps you came back from an injury and you used imagery to 'pace' yourself and manage your expectations. Or you felt a bit overwhelmed by playing a super important match and you imagined being in a quiet place, like a nice beach or forest, to calm yourself down. Or you went through which serve to play next in a badminton match. Now let's move from sport to labour. What are some reasons that you can think about that you could use imagery for? Maybe you could use it to feel more confident, manage pain and imagine the contractions as waves that move out of the body, or to stay patient.

So far, you have read about what imagery is and what the different components of imagery are. You may have also started to think about what you can use imagery for. Now, how can we combine this so that imagery can be used as a purposeful strategy? First, it is helpful to consider what the purpose of using the imagery is, do you need it to give you the motivation to push through when you are tired and in pain or discomfort, or to help you pace yourself when you are fed up with waiting for the contractions to become more regular? Do you want to use imagery to help with confidence and your belief that you can do it? Do you want to use imagery to help you to try to stay calm and feel more relaxed? Do you want to use it as a pain management tool? Or perhaps you could use imagery to help with breathing techniques. There are lots of different uses for imagery, but you may just want to focus on the ones that you feel are most important and meaningful to you, as otherwise, it is easy to get overwhelmed. It may well be that using imagery to feel calm helps you to manage your pain, and that's all you need it for! I will give a few examples of how imagery can be used for feeling relaxed, motivation and pacing, pain management confidence/self-belief, and birthing technique below.

A very popular use of imagery in general and during labour is to feel more relaxed and reduce the pressure you may be feeling. In fact, a lot of guided imagery intends to put someone in a state of relaxation. This has a lot of benefits – if you feel (mental)pressure, this can affect the release of 'fight or flight' related hormones such as cortisol. Focusing on feeling relaxed and decreasing muscle tension can help to reduce these cortisol levels. An example of how you can do this is to think about a 'happy' place. What is a place that makes you feel relaxed and calm? For some this could be somewhere in nature, like the sea and the sound of the waves or the mountains, and for others it may be having a good time with friends or listening to calming music. You can also try to imagine the muscle tension leaving your body with every breath you take. Whatever it is, make sure that it is personal to you, and that it is not too stimulating, as that then has the effect that you get overly excited!

You can also use imagery to help you get in a positive mood state. This is often done in combination with relaxation imagery, but this does not necessarily have to be the case. You can draw from positive past experiences, perhaps a good and enjoyable sport performance, to help you get in a positive mood. This can be particularly relevant in the lead-up to labour, as well as those very early stages of labour where levels of oxytocin are helpful. Getting yourself in a positive mood state will help you to move away from feeling anxious and stressed, and you could visualise times where endorphins were high, similar to that feeling after a great workout or that runner's high feeling. Having music in the background that reminds you of an enjoyable time can be a useful tool to support re-creating positive previous experiences in your mind. Just remember that as you progress through the stages of labour that these can have very different demands and being adaptable is so important.

The lead-up to giving birth can be hard work. You may have been waiting for this for a long time, and the last couple of weeks can be very tiring, where it may feel a bit like running out of gas. Motivation is such an intriguing concept, which is all about what drives you. The fascinating thing about motivation is that you can have a lot of motivation but not always for the best reason, that is, the quantity of motivation can be high, but the quality less so. Typically, 'high' quality motivation is motivation that comes from within and is within your control, that is, you are doing something or engaging in an activity because you want it, not because others are dictating it. In sport psychology (and lots of other fields of psychology!) this is called intrinsic motivation. If you are motivated to do something because you feel pressure to do so or are being told by others that it would be good for you to do, then this is usually extrinsic motivation. The reason that I would classify this as lower-quality motivation is because extrinsic motivation is controlled by external factors, and as such it can cause a lot of pressure. Research also consistently finds that intrinsic motivation has better well-being outcomes compared to extrinsic motivation. This is, however, not to say that extrinsic motivation is always bad! It does serve a function and can give you that extra push to keep you going. For me thinking about eating some camembert and sushi was quite a nice extrinsic motivator in the hours before being induced, but admittedly this was the last thing on my mind after the contractions had properly kicked in! In essence, it is all about having an understanding of what informs your motivation, and to make sure that you are not solely driven by external factors that can affect your well-being in a negative way. In an ideal world, you want to have a lot (high quantity) of intrinsic (high quality) motivation.

That was a bit of a sidestep to explain motivation, let's get back on track to how you can use imagery to feel more motivated (whichever type of motivation you feel you need at the time). For example, you may be strongly motivated by the moment that you have the first skin-to-skin contact with your baby. In the moment, you are feeling tired and struggling to keep up with the contractions. You can use the image of what it feels like to push the baby out as motivation throughout the different stages of labour. Imagine that every contraction moves the baby further down the birth canal, drawing on all your senses, and use this as motivation to take it one contraction at the time, and pace yourself. This is something that you can practice in the lead-up to labour, perhaps using different images and videos, so that it becomes easier to use imagery when you are in the moment and feeling tired. Maybe (a bit of an extrinsic reward!) you imagine that nice meal after the labour, and use this as motivation to keep calm when the birth is not going as expected. Pip (midwife and runner) suggested that women can pack two jars, one empty and one filled with sweets, for every contraction you, or your birth partner, move one sweet to the empty jar. This is a nice way of combining chunking (from the goal-setting chapter) with imagery. Seeing these jars fill up can be a visual way of seeing yourself progressing through labour, and you can use this to imagine that every single contraction is productive, you can tick that one off, and you are getting one step closer to meeting the baby. What is helpful when you are using imagery to help you with motivation is to be aware of what drives you, and use this to subsequently inform your imagery when you feel you are running out of energy.

Getting yourself in a relaxed and positive emotional state can be beneficial when it comes to pain management. As mentioned earlier, being in a relaxed state can help to manage excessive levels of stress hormones; remember that having too high levels of stress hormones can make pain feel more intense. In general, research has found that using imagery can reduce or reframe the pain, and this is probably one of the most popular uses of imagery when it comes to labour. One way to use imagery for pain management is that you can use imagery to start seeing pain as something that is *not* uncontrollable. For example, you can decide to breathe into the pain and really tune in to the pain. Perhaps you can imagine that the pain is a shape, and that you change it from a square into a circle, or see it as a wave that exits the body and helps to move you one step closer to meeting the baby. Another way you can see the pain as something you can have a sense of control over is to think about the purpose the pain has, which can be combined with reflecting on your motivation as described above; if you are having a vaginal birth, with every contraction, the baby descends down the birth canal. It is a bit like a step-by-step approach, as illustrated by Amy (skeleton): 'The pain is because you are giving birth, and giving birth is because you want to see your baby and then your baby is out in the world. So it is just that step by step. I have to have the pain, I have to have the contractions, because I have to push, because I have to get the baby out, and I can't wait to see the baby'. Imagining that your body is moving oxygen around and working with the baby can be a powerful narrative for this and that the pain is a positive aspect of the process. You can also imagine yourself as a strong ship wading through high waves; this can not only help with pain management but also give yourself confidence. One mother I interviewed, Paola, a Crossfit trainer who teaches women during and post pregnancy, explained that after each contraction, she visualised that she had wiped another contraction off the table, and this would give her the confidence to keep going.

Women have also used imagery to move their attention away from the pain, like dimming or switching off the light, to use an analogy. Moving your attention away from the pain can be achieved by redirecting your focus from the pain to how powerful your body is and to really breathe into the contractions. You can combine this with positive affirmations (covered more in the next chapter), such as 'with every breath I keep the baby happy, and we are one step closer to meeting each other'. If the situation enables this, you can combine this imagery with movements that mimic the movements of the baby. Using imagery to move your attention away from the pain can also be done through imagining that you are in a different place, perhaps a nice scenic destination, or through imagining another activity that you enjoy doing. Be careful, however, not to use this dissociative imagery all the time. When you think about a happy place or a relaxed beach, this can give temporary relief, but sometimes tuning in to the pain and discomfort can help to understand what your body is going through and how to manage this. It can also help with communicating any potentially worrisome pain signals to the team around you, which you may ignore if you just focus on using dissociative imagery to move away from the pain you experience in your body.

Imagery is also a powerful tool to help you feel confident. Remember that in chapter 2, I spoke about how recalling previous successful experiences can help to inform your self-belief, as well as seeing other people in a similar situation being successful. Together, these sources can be used to help (re)create powerful experiences to give you confidence. As there might be some unexpected experiences during labour that you have not experienced before, you can start by recalling a time where you managed to deal with a difficult situation in a confident manner. This may have been a time at work or when you were playing your sport. Recall how your body felt and what emotions you experienced. Reliving those can help you to create a strong vision of yourself. Imagine that good things will happen or that you are able to manage unexpected situations in a confident way. Imagining being successful when you may struggle can be really powerful and may have a calming effect. Again, it is important to practice this in the lead-up to labour, so that it is much easier to draw on this as a tool.

If you are giving birth in a medical setting, some women feel they are lacking confidence when surrounded by medical professionals in an environment they are unfamiliar with. In one of my birth preparation classes, we mimicked a caesarean birth scenario where the women were asked to act out different members of the team, such as the midwife, consultant obstetrician, anaesthetist, paediatrician, obstetrician's assistant, scrub nurse, theatre nurses, and the birth partner (if allowed to be present). I found this helpful as I had not quite realised how crowded the operation theatre would be; this helped me to then imagine what the situation could be like, even though this was a scenario that was very much a scenario I did not prefer (but I knew that it was not something that would be within my control). Using imagery to create and think about the different options offered to you can be helpful in the decision-making processes. This is something that does need practice, and you may be able to draw on your sporting experiences where you imagined different pacing strategies when you were cycling, or perhaps you imagined a change from one defensive tactic to another in football, or had a difficult conversation about your training schedule with your coach. More importantly, ensuring that you have the relevant information accessible to you, perhaps through educational sessions, antenatal classes or reading about scenarios relevant to your situation, is helpful to imagine the different options available to you. You can also imagine the medical staff as being part of your support team, if that's something you find helpful. If you have given birth before, you can also draw on the (positive) experiences of your first birth.

Another purpose of using imagery during labour is to imagine your birthing technique. This may be the positions that you are looking to use during the different phases of giving birth or to imagine the muscles that you need to use when pushing the baby out. The latter example is particularly relevant to practice in the lead-up to giving birth if you have planned to get an epidural as part of your birth plan. Alda, who played tennis in college, and who lives in California, requested an epidural for both her children. She explained that, although she knew she wanted an epidural, she had not considered to practice which muscles to use when pushing the baby out. As she could not feel anything, she felt that she ended up pushing too hard with her first child, resulting in haemorrhoids that were very painful. With her second child, she made sure to practice which muscles to use when pushing, and to just focus on these, rather than the whole body. Although she could not feel the sensations after she had the epidural, she used imagery to focus her pushing efforts on the uterus muscles and pushed in a more controlled rather than all-out effort. She did not suffer from haemorrhoids this time. This is such a powerful illustration of how imagery can work, and even if you don't have an epidural in your birth plan, you may end up with one, so it's worth learning how to use the 'pushing' muscles. You can speak with health practitioners, doulas, midwives and mothers to help you understand which muscles are involved to help you create a vivid image and help you during the pushing stage. An example of how you can use imagery during the first stage of labour was given by Pip (midwife, runner). To help support physical changes that are happening at this stage, where the cervix is pulled upwards into the sides of the uterus, causing the cervix to open up or dilate, she used an 'upward breath and visualisation'. She did this by visualising a giant yellow balloon in her abdomen and pelvic area, deflated to start off with, and when a contraction came, she would breathe upwards and imagine that yellow balloon filling up with air and floating up to fill up her entire abdomen. This helped her to focus on her breathing and took her mind away from everything else that was going on around her.

Using imagery as a tool

So how to go from here and have imagery as a tool during labour? The first step you have already taken, that is to learn what imagery is, perhaps you have reflected on how you have used it before, and you have an idea of what the different uses are. The next step is to get familiar with using imagery in a more purposeful manner using some of the information that I covered above to strengthen your imagery skills. In the lemon script you have already started to consider a few aspects of imagery, such as using your senses to enhance vividness of the image and the controllability of the image. Once you are ready to start with imagery, find yourself a quiet and calm place, so that you won't be distracted, and take a few deep breaths. After you have practiced using imagery a few times, you will find that you are able to apply imagery in places where there might be some distractions. This is quite important to have practiced, as you don't always have the opportunity to control the environment that you are giving birth in. There may be some distractions such as sounds or bright lights, and having practiced imagery beforehand in an environment with some distractions will then make you feel more confident that you can use it in other environments with some distractions. This has of course also the advantage that you can tune in to using imagery to distance yourself from some of the distractions, such as a busy labour ward, and to keep calm. This brings us to the next step of how to use imagery and identify what you want to use it for. What is the purpose of using imagery, what do you want to use it for in the birthing process? Is it to stay calm and positive? For pain management? To fuel your energy when you feel you've run out of steam?

To summarise, these are the three points I just described.

1. Understand what imagery is
2. Familiarise yourself with imagery – start with basic scripts
3. Identify what you want to use the imagery for

Imagery is not one of the easiest sport psychology strategies to get your head around. You may have found it a bit difficult to generate the lemon image or found it challenging to control it. How can you get better at creating an image and feel that you have control over it? Although we use imagery all the time, it can be difficult to use imagery in this purposeful manner. Quite often we lose control over the images or can't get a clear or vivid image. Just like the other strategies, it is important to train imagery.

Layered stimulus response training

One approach to developing your imagery skills is called layered stimulus-response training. This approach focuses on breaking down the image first and then slowly building up the image again. This way you learn to have more control over the image and find it easier to create images when you need them. Let's have a look at this in a bit more detail.

Images can have different elements; in technical terms, these are typically called stimulus, response, and meaning propositions. A stimulus proposition has to do with the situation, so this can be where you'd give birth (hospital, home, birth centre), the people who would be there, sounds and so on. Response propositions are your response to that situation; you can think about your heart beating in your throat, tense muscles, or relaxed breathing. Response propositions also include your emotions; maybe the stimulus situation triggers happy feelings, or feeling tense or scared. The meaning proposition is about how you interpret these response propositions; do you see it as something that is helpful, like a positive challenge, or as something that is unhelpful, a negative threat?

Knowing about these three elements is useful because this will help you to create an image, which is the first step of layered stimulus-response training. You start with a basic image that you will build up in a way to help you achieve your goal, or intended image, for example to stay calm in a pressurised situation. Think about the situation you want to develop the imagery for, such as imagining packing your hospital bag, or imagining yourself getting ready to serve in tennis. As this is the first layer, you want to draw from a situation that you are familiar with. Once you have identified the situation, you describe it out loud, where is it, when is it, what is it? Then you close your eyes and imagine the situation in your mind.

When you have finished imagining the situation, you rate the vividness and the clarity of the image. You can do this on a 5-point scale (1 = no image to 5 = a clear and vivid image) as we did after the lemon script. In addition to the vividness, you can also reflect on how much control you had over the image, whether you felt any changes in your heart rate or muscle tension and so on. This is what is called the reflection stage of the layered stimulus-response training. If you feel that you find it difficult to create a vivid image or find it hard to control the image, then you stick with the image and practice again.

If you feel that the basic image is clear and controllable, you can add a layer to it by adding more detail to the content of the image. Perhaps you start to imagine traveling to the hospital. You will then engage in the reflection stage again before adding another layer of detail to the image. If the image, and in particular the meaning propositions, turns negative and you feel you constantly lose control over the image, then you might find it useful to have a conversation with someone about why that may be the case. If you have not used imagery as a strategy before whilst playing your sport, or in other domains, remember that you do not have to use imagery as a technique for labour if you are not comfortable using it.

The first layer of layered stimulus-response training is often based on your personal experience as it can be easier to recall these. If this is the first time you are giving birth, there will be a whole bunch of unknowns. Of course, you can't prepare for everything, but there are some things that you could do to help creating vivid (and I'd like to emphasise realistic and helpful) images in your mind. I can still vividly remember one of my appointments in the birth centre, where a powerful and primal sound appeared from one of the rooms. It was such an intense sound and it helped to prepare me for what was to come, and I could create an image of a primal sound in my head, without feeling scared or intimidated by the sound. Watching it on TV is not quite the same! It also helped me to normalise this sound and to not feel bothered or self-conscious in case I would make a sound like this myself. Moreover, it made me feel so empowered; she sounded so powerful!

If there is an opportunity for you to have a tour of the birth or labour room (even if it is a virtual one), go for it. When you visit these places, use all your senses to really take in the experiences. You can focus on the smells, the sounds, the lights, the temperature and so on. Using all your senses can help you to create that vivid experience of what the birth room or labour ward feels like, which may help you to mentally prepare for the different things that can happen and enable you to stay calm when things do not go to plan. If it is allowed, do bring your birth partner with you. You may also want to consider that even though you are planning to give birth in a particular place, like the birth centre, to also look at the labour ward. This may make it easier if you have to throw overboard your birth plan, as you already have imagined what the labour room would look like, or the operating theatre for a C-section. It all becomes a lot less intimidating this way. I would like to reiterate the importance of realistic images that are in line with your situation. It's not helpful to create an image of you giving birth at home in a pool with candles, lavender scent and calm music if realistically you know that you'd feel more comfortable in a hospital environment or that a lavender scent or music are going to irritate you after a while. Similarly, only imagining 'doom' scenarios is not going to benefit your confidence and psychological well-being.

Take-home message

1. How can imagery help you to approach the maternity journey as a positive challenge? For example, using imagery to visualise how to push indicates an approach focus (what you intend to do), imagining that you are physically strong can give you self-belief, and using imagery to focus on breathing techniques can help you to focus on something that is within your control.

2. There are many reasons why you could use imagery; remember that you don't need to use it for everything. If imagining a happy place helps you to engage with your breathing and to stay calm, then that may be all that is needed for you at that moment in time.

3. Imagery may take a bit of practice, yet it can be a very useful tool in the lead-up and during labour. After reading this chapter, you may even have realised that you are already using it and can add it to your toolbox with perhaps some more practice. To remind yourself to keep developing your imagery, you can identify some cues related to everyday tasks that can serve as reminders to engage in imagery.

4. If you have identified a particular reason or scenario to use imagery for, you could consider recording an imagery script and listen to this regularly to help you strengthen your imagery.

5. Most people can relate to times when they used strategies to deal with situations, but we often do not make the connection to how to use these strategies in a different context, like in labour. If you feel that imagery is too much for you to use as a tool, then don't feel you need to. Remember that you decide which tools you want to fill your toolbox with.

6 'I got this': Self-talk as a strategy in your toolkit

We constantly talk to ourselves. How many thoughts we have per day exactly we don't quite know, yet with estimates varying from 6,000 to 80,000 thoughts per day, that is a lot of chatter going on in our mind! A lot of these thoughts are automatic and repetitive. We don't really notice or pay much attention to these, and are often not really aware of what we are saying to ourselves. As such, what you sometimes want to do is to listen to your thoughts to become more aware of what this chatter in your mind is about. When you begin to pay attention to some of these thoughts, you start to notice that these are not always that helpful. Whereas that may not be news to you, and the last thing you want to do is to tune in to these negative, or unhelpful, thoughts all the time, you do need to become aware of them if you do not want to let these unhelpful thoughts get to you and take over.

When you think about your involvement in sport, you may recall situations when the negative and unhelpful thoughts took over. Perhaps you told yourself that your teammates would be upset and that you'd be a failure if you missed that penalty shot late in a game, or you said to yourself that you're stupid for hitting the tennis ball wide. Or you had the thought that your legs will never be able to get you up the hill when you were doing a hill rep training session, or that you wanted to give up and go home around mile 22 in a marathon. All those thoughts are not particularly helpful, but so common! When I work with sportspeople, a lot of the work focuses on exploring these thoughts and to understand why these can have such an influence on not just performance but also on how sport is experienced. Having a lot of negative and unhelpful thoughts like these can really take the enjoyment factor out of sports. Although it is not realistic to say that you can eradicate negative thoughts, there are tools, such as using strategic self-talk, that can be used to help manage some of these thoughts.

In this chapter, I will cover the usefulness of self-talk, where some of this self-talk may come from, as well as provide some tips on how you can use self-talk as a tool. I have given some examples of self-talk in sport settings, but of course in the lead-up to labour and during labour, a lot of thoughts will go through your mind. Some of these tend to be more helpful than others. Have a read through the examples below; which of these would you label as unhelpful self-talk and why?

- I can't do this any longer, what am I doing here?
- The baby must come out now, I can't bear it any longer
- I am only dilated 2 cm; this is going to take ages
- I got this; I know it is going to hurt, but my body is ready for it, and so am I
- This pain is something else, come on, you can do it!

During my pregnancy, I went to some antenatal yoga classes that were delivered by a very experienced doula. Although we did a bit of antenatal yoga, most of the time, she shared her stories with us, and these were invaluable in helping me prepare for the journey ahead. One thing that she kept coming back to in her stories was that a lot of women focus on how much they are dilated, and that when this is assessed, and it is not as far progressed as they thought it should be, there was a real sense of disappointment. This disappointment could then really take them out of their bubble and stall the progress. As such, telling yourself that you are *only* dilated 2 centimetres is not that helpful. Your body is doing a great job, and everyone progresses at their own pace. Yes, perhaps it may take a bit longer for your body than someone else, but if the situation is safe and the baby is happy, then there is no need to tell yourself that it is *only* 2 cm (or whichever number you had in mind). What is much more useful is to use self-talk that directs you back on the road ahead and keeps you in that zone.

So, what can make some of these thoughts unhelpful? Firstly, some thoughts can be unhelpful because they are very rigid. Thoughts or statements like 'I *must* give birth naturally', or 'It would be *awful* if my baby is in a complete breech position', 'A c-section is out of the question and not an option' are examples of rigid thoughts. Of course, it may not be what you have hoped for, but it does not have to be the end of the world. In labour, rigid thoughts can be unhelpful as there is so much in labour that is out of one's control. Adding a layer of rigid thoughts to an experience that already requires so much physical, physiological, and mental effort can make it even harder. Rigid thoughts are often linked to irrational beliefs, which can also lead to unhelpful behaviours such as avoidance. I will get back to 'irrational beliefs' a bit later in this chapter when we go through some examples of how you can use something called rational emotive behaviour therapy (REBT) to manage these negative thoughts.

Quite a few of the examples I have given so far are thoughts that tend to pop up spontaneously in our mind; these thoughts are not necessarily regulated. These are examples of spontaneously talking to yourself, and sometimes you may feel that you do not have full control over this spontaneous chatter. To help you change how to use or manage your thoughts in a more helpful way, there are a few different approaches you could take.

Let's have a look at strategic, or intentional, self-talk first. Intentional self-talk is where you plan to use self-talk, often in a systematic way. When I work with sportspeople on their use of self-talk, the first step is to become aware of some of their (recurring) spontaneous thoughts and reflect on how useful these thoughts are. After this reflection, we work on strategies to help manage these thoughts; this can be to accept thoughts for what they are and let the thoughts 'just be' (see chapter 7/8 for some examples of how to do this), and/or to introduce more purposeful and intentional use of self-talk where we work on self-talk statements that are useful for them. What I do not tend to do, however, is to work with people on suppressing the thoughts, as this can take a lot of energy. And of course, if through the reflection we find out that there is a lot of helpful self-talk, then the focus is on using these when they play their sports. You can't manage or change every single thought after all; imagine doing this with all those thousand thoughts every day! When we do work on intentional self-talk statements, the focus of these statements can be on managing unhelpful thoughts, to increase motivation, pacing, focus on the process, to feel more confident and so on. In sport psychology, we tend to distinguish between instructional and motivational self-talk. Although there is often overlap, it can be quite helpful to look at these in turn to get an insight into how you can use intentional self-talk.

We will start with instructional self-talk, which is self-talk used to provide guidance or instruction related to a task; this can be technique or form, strategy, and what to focus on. It can help us to keep our focus on the process. If we take swimming, having a good breathing technique is an integral part and you'd like to make sure that every breath counts. Having a rhythm helps. As such, an example of instructional self-talk is that every time you take a breath, you tell yourself to exhale the moment your face touches the water.

Of course, breathing is very important in labour. Talking yourself through controlled breathing can help to give you ownership and make you feel that you are in control. Ways of doing this could be counting, focusing on posture, and active birth movements. It can also help to make you feel confident and inform your self-belief. Here is an example: 'deep breathe in, fill my lungs with air, so that I am ready for a powerful contraction'. Whatever the instruction is, make sure that it is a short one, as otherwise you might be overloading your mind.

Other ways you can use instructional self-talk is to help with pacing. A lot of runners I have worked with at mass participation events tend to race off at the start and throw their pacing plan overboard as they get carried away in the moment. Having an instructional self-talk statement such as 'steady does it', 'go at my own pace' can all be helpful to not get carried away at the start and focus on the process, which in this instance is their pacing strategy. When we consider labour, pacing is definitely a factor. This can be seen by counting the time between contractions or to pace yourself through the different intensity phases of a contraction. Wanting to go too fast or push too early can be harmful, and a helpful instructional self-talk statement in this instance could be 'one contraction at a time', or 'don't get ahead of myself, when the baby is ready I can start to push'.

Instructional self-talk can also be used to give you confidence, you can use self-talk to remind yourself of a time where you have successfully managed a similar situation. Using instructional self-talk can also be very helpful to remind you to relax your body. Just telling yourself to relax is probably not going to be as helpful, and could even be a bit stressful as you are well aware of the need for a relaxed body! Instead, you can use a more specific instructional self-talk statement such as 'soften your shoulders' or 'let's melt into the bed and soften up my body'.

Motivational self-talk is the use of self-talk for, and the name gives it away, motivational purposes. This type of intentional self-talk is less about the process and more about encouragement and cheering yourself on. Examples of motivational self-talk are: 'You are doing a great job', 'You're strong, keep going!'. This type of self-talk is especially helpful when you might feel you are getting low on energy. You can imagine that motivational self-talk is a big factor during child birth, especially considering the energy and effort that it requires when the labour is taking quite a long time. You may feel that you are running out of steam, and motivational self-talk can help to re-energise. You could also draw on inspirational others to give you that confidence and motivation for a final push, for example, 'Many others have succeeded before me, I am strong and confident and I will find the power to push'.

Intentional self-talk can be used on its own or together with other strategies. From my work with athletes, I know that the strategies covered in this book are often used together and that they can complement each other. An example is to combine instructional self-talk with imagery, where you can talk yourself through what it looks like to release the tension in your body. Another example could be that you tell yourself that through the process of contractions, you are making room for the baby to come out, and together with telling yourself this, you can imagine the cervix widening to make space for your baby. A way of combining intentional self-talk with goal-setting and focus on the process could be to keep your eyes on the road by drawing on a self-talk statement like 'one contraction at the time'. What this illustrates is that you can easily combine the different strategies in the book and use these together, even though it might not always be that obvious.

Making an impact with self-talk

When considering using self-talk as a strategy, two things are important to start with. First, you want to gain an insight into what you are saying to yourself; this is important before you can start to do something about it. Second, you want to think about what you want to use self-talk for. It can be related to finding energy to keep going, managing emotions, or feeling confident. Below I give two examples of approaches you can take, the IMPACT approach and rational emotive behaviour therapy (REBT). The IMPACT approach is a proactive approach to use intentional self-talk, and REBT is about reflecting on your thoughts and disputing beliefs that are unhelpful or irrational and optimising performance beliefs. I also briefly touch on positive affirmations.

One approach that has been used in endurance sport settings to develop a self-talk strategy, and integrates becoming aware of your self-talk and considering your reasons for using self-talk is the IMPACT approach. IMPACT stands for: I (identify what you want to achieve), M (match self-talk to your needs), P (practice different cues with consistency), A (ascertain which cues work best for you), C (create specific self-talk plans), T (train self-talk plans to perfection).

The first step is to **identify** the goal, what is it that you want to achieve? Let's say that what you want to achieve is to stay calm and let go of controlling the uncontrollable when things do not go according to plan. I realise that especially for first-time mothers, it can be difficult to know what it is that you want to achieve. It is also a very personal thing, yet you can have conversations with others about this and then reflect on what would be helpful for you.

The second step is to **match** self-talk to your needs. For example, if you know that you find it difficult to focus when you are in pain, then you want to come up with some self-talk statements that help you to tune back in to the 'zone'. It may be that this is a combination of motivational and instructional self-talk statements. See below for some examples of matching self-talk to your needs.

Need	Example of self-talk statement
Feeling out of control – focus on breathing to regain attention	Slow breath in, pause for a second, slow breath out. Let's keep a rhythm. *This is a time where instructional self-talk can be quite useful to help guide your breathing or remind you of breathing techniques.*
Managing pain	Wow, this hurts! Okay, I know that the pain is part of the process. Let's play (happy song) in my head to take my mind off it for a minute. *This is a situation where you can't just ignore that you are having the thought that it hurts. You can use a subsequent statement to redirect your thoughts.*
Feeling frustrated and inpatient / running out of steam	Come on, you can do this, just focus on one step at a time. *This is a situation where motivational self-talk can be useful to help keep the momentum going.*
Your examples!	

The third step is to **practice** your self-talk statements. This can be a rather tricky one, as you won't be able to practice giving birth and then try out the self-talk statements. But what you can do is find situations that are (somewhat) similar to what it is that you want to achieve. For example, if the goal is to tune in to pain, are there any (safe) situations where you can practice this? Here is an example that may be useful: A few years ago, I started to dip my toes in trying out yoga. I had mostly avoided yoga up to that point as I felt that I was so inflexible and could not bear the thought of standing next to a yogi and feeling utterly incompetent! Anyway, I got over that and found a brilliant yoga class. I vividly remember one of the first sessions where I learned about the 'pigeon' position. Wow, did that hurt my stiff hips! After the initial shock of how long a minute could feel, I started to use (instructional) self-talk to help me focus on my breathing and later to help me tune in to the pain. Over time, this really helped me to use self-talk as a pain management tool. I did make sure though to check whether it was 'good' or 'bad' pain. Over the years, I have had too many times that I was silly enough to play through injury (bad pain) where I should have really rested up. So, during my pregnancy, I used an adapted pigeon pose to help me practice my self-talk to help manage the discomfort. I used statements such as 'the pain is temporary', and I varied this with counting to help my mind distract from the discomfort.

This practice is really important, so that you have a chance to reflect on the statements. After you have practiced your self-talk statements, you want to **ascertain** which ones worked for you. This can be done through reflection questions such as:

- Which self-talk statements did I use?
- How easy was it to use the self-talk statement?
- How did I feel about using this statement?
- Was the self-talk statement helpful? Why and how?

If there are any statements, however, that make you feel tenser or more agitated, or confused, then it is probably a good time to disregard these and focus on the self-talk statements that you can relate to and that you feel that you can remember and use in the lead-up and during labour. Make a note of these and use these to **create** your self-talk plan.

Based on the above, you can select a few statements that you want to take with you into the labour room, at home or wherever you give birth. You may find a table like the one below useful to guide your self-talk plan.

Stage of labour	What is the need? What do you want to use the self-talk for?	What is a self-talk statement that would be useful for you?
Mid-labour	Managing contractions	It's a wave flowing through my body, getting the baby closer one contraction at a time.

Finally, you want to **train** the self-talk plan. Of course, you cannot practice labour, but there are plenty of occasions where you can practice self-talk. For example, if you are working during your pregnancy, there may be times at work when you feel frustrated and you can then train the self-talk statements to help you stay calm; for example, through a statement reminding yourself to focus on calm breathing. Similarly, if you are still able to do exercise, you can use self-talk to help with pacing or to focus on postures when doing strength exercises, all of which can help in labour.

Positive affirmations

Before I move on to managing irrational thoughts, I want to briefly touch on *positive affirmations.* Some of what I explained above is not too dissimilar to having a positive affirmation, which is something that is often covered in hypnobirthing. It is great to have a bank of positive affirmations available to you, but it is important that you find affirmations that work for you and that you can relate to. It is not helpful to use positive affirmations like 'I quiet my mind and let my body give birth' when you feel like your mind is in overdrive, you have worries about how the labour is progressing and don't know how to calm down. A more specific instructional self-talk statement focused on how to calm down can be more useful in this instance. Also, don't try to have too many statements, as it will be difficult to remember all of them. I can't emphasise enough how important autonomy is here too. Using self-talk statements that are meaningful to you and that you have come up with, or chosen, have much more of an effect than self-talk statements that you have been told to use or that you are using because someone else used them. It is much harder to remember the self-talk statements in this latter case. Whatever your self-talk statements are, it is important that you practice, adapt, and practice some more so that the statements are easily accessible to you.

If you can use positive affirmations to get you in a rhythm, then that can be helpful too. Affirmations can be especially helpful in letting you switch off the busy brain and don't let all these thoughts take over. It is really hard to say two different things to yourself at the same time – so a positive affirmation can be great in taking you away from any worrying thoughts you may have and allowing you to focus on the process of birth. As such, it is important that you have some brief and simple statements that are easy to remember and help you to focus on the task (whichever stage of labour you are in). Some examples of popular affirmations are: 'I trust my body', 'My baby will come out', 'The pain helps to move the baby out', 'I am strong', 'We are a team'. Have you thought about any affirmations? You can write these down and pick the top ones that you can relate to.

Using the self-talk statements in labour

Once you have established self-talk statements as part of the IMPACT approach or identified positive affirmations that are meaningful to you, you can share these with your birth partner, so that they can remind you of them. Do make sure that your birth partner is also aware of when to stay quiet, and of what not to say, as there have been plenty of women who just want their partner to 'shut up' because of well-intended but not so useful verbal encouragement. Preparing them beforehand will also prevent you from getting upset or frustrated with their well-intended words of encouragement when all you need them to do is stay quiet!

You can write your statements down if you find that helpful, and hang them on the wall or somewhere where you can see them (if you manage to keep your eyes open!). If you are in a labour room, midwives or the obstetrician might be happy for you to do this, although there is not always time or space to do this. You may also find it helpful to write down your mantra or statements in your birth plan and, dependable on your midwife or obstetrician, the relationship with them and the labour situation, they may remind you of these at various stages of the labour.

Quite a few women I spoke to were not aware of whether they were using self-talk statements during their labour, yet when they were sharing their birth story, it was evident that they drew on instructional self-talk to talk themselves through breathing strategies. Others used motivational self-talk at stages of labour when they needed to energise themselves or feel strong. One of the women reflected on how she used the statement 'powerful hero', and how she had never felt so strong in her life up to that moment. This is really fascinating, and what this shows to me is that we are not always aware of how we may be using a lot of the strategies that we have available to us. It emphasises the importance of reflecting on how we can learn from other situations that we have experienced and use these reflections to help give us the confidence that we have more strategies available to us than we initially thought. Of course, also remember to keep practicing the statements, so that it is easier to implement their use!

Managing irrational thoughts

We will now move from intentional self-talk statements to REBT, which is more about managing unhelpful chatter in our heads. At the start of this chapter, I asked you to think about the usefulness of statements such as 'the baby must come out now, I *can't bear it any longer*' and 'I am only dilated 2 cm, this is going to take ages, and *this is terrible*', which can be labelled as irrational beliefs. Irrational beliefs can be rather detrimental because they are rigid, demanding and sometimes those beliefs might feel as if it's the end of the world. Irrational beliefs cannot be 'true' because they are not based on reality. For example, the thought that you are only dilated 2 cm is not irrational itself, but the belief that it is terrible can turn it into an irrational belief. Telling yourself that you can't stand something is also unhelpful as it makes the discomfort associated with what you can't stand even stronger. A lot of irrational beliefs result in avoidance behaviours; this can be wanting to take yourself out of the situation mentally, such as switching off and not taking anything in, or physically, such as wanting to walk away, or a combination of physical and mental avoidance. Irrational beliefs can also fuel unhelpful emotions such as anxiety. The take-away message here is that generally irrational beliefs are not particularly helpful, yet irrational thoughts are pretty common. So what can we do to shift irrational beliefs to more rational beliefs? This is where REBT can be helpful.

In recent years, REBT has gained popularity in sport psychology. REBT is helpful when trying to understand how we work by looking at thoughts, emotions, and behaviours. REBT is, simply said, about questioning the *belief* you have about something, like a situation, and to become more flexible and rational in your thinking. Where the self-talk strategy of using intentional self-talk statements, covered earlier in the chapter, is mostly about using a statement to help guide your actions, such as breathing or to help with motivation, REBT is about reflecting on what you are saying to yourself and to dispute, or question, beliefs that are irrational. What is central to REBT is that it is not the emotion ('I am upset and disappointed') that you are questioning, nor the event itself, but it is the belief ('I completely forgot how to breathe properly, therefore I am such a failure') that you focus on. This focus on the thought or belief is what makes it relevant to consider in this chapter because you can then use more rational thoughts as self-talk statements. As you may recall from earlier in the book, our thoughts have a powerful influence on our emotions and our behaviour. Rational beliefs can lead to more of an approach focus where you want to tackle the situation 'head on', and take appropriate action (which can sometimes be a deliberate decision of 'inaction'!). As a recap, what is important to remember when it comes to REBT is that it is not the emotion that you are questioning, but it is the thought, or belief, that you focus on. Doing so could help you to decrease emotional distress and engage in less self-defeating behaviours, such as sticking your head in the sand or becoming overly tense.

Although this might sound rather easy, by no means am I suggesting this to be the case, as the intricacies of REBT can get a bit complicated. We won't get into the nitty-gritty of it in this book, but if the information in this chapter can help you become more aware of irrational beliefs and helps you to draw on more rational beliefs, then that is a great takeaway. If you want help with disputing your irrational thoughts, you can look for someone specialised in REBT to help you with this. REBT is also a useful approach to take to help you with focus on the here and now, which can be rather helpful when it comes to labour. I talk more about focus in Chapter 8, so let's now have a brief look at how REBT works.

How to do REBT

To manage irrational beliefs, let's have a look at what is called the 'GABCDE model'. This model is a way to help you find out where the irrational beliefs are coming from as well as dispute these beliefs. This is done by considering the **G**oals, **A**ctivating events, **B**eliefs and **C**onsequences, followed by **D**isputing the irrational beliefs and **E**ffective new beliefs.

The **A**ctivating event is what you feel is the adverse or negative event. This does not have to be something that has just happened; it can also be something that might happen in the future, or it might be something that you imagine might happen. To get a picture of the activating event, you want to ask yourself questions about what happened in the situation, followed by asking yourself what you made of the situation. What was it about the perceived adversity or event that made you feel stressed, uncomfortable or led you to do something that was not particularly helpful? What is it about the event that made it hinder your **G**oals?

When you are exploring the Activating event, you may start to think about how you respond to the event in terms of your feelings (emotions), your actions (behaviour), and your thoughts. This is what is called the **C**onsequences in REBT. You want to spend a little bit of time exploring your thoughts, behaviours, and feelings, so that you can create a fuller picture of the consequences. It can be quite common to think that these consequences alone are a direct result of the event; this is not what REBT is about. It is the **B**elief about the event that leads to the feelings, behaviours, and thoughts.

Let's explore this a bit further. Irrational beliefs are often fuelled by **B**eliefs that things must be in a certain way, like a demand, as well as beliefs such as I can't stand it when things don't go my way, it is the end of the world when I don't live up to these standards, and I am worthless if I can't do it. All of these are not particularly helpful, can even be unhealthy, yet we sometimes accept these beliefs without critiquing them. The idea of REBT is to learn to replace these irrational beliefs with more healthy beliefs or weaken the irrational beliefs and to make the rational beliefs stronger. This is where the next step, disputing the irrational thoughts come in.

Disputing irrational thoughts can be done by asking questions about how logical, realistic, and pragmatic the belief is. You can consider the questions below as a guide for this.

- How logical is the belief?
  - Does it seem logical that I 'must' do this?
  - Does it make sense?
  - Is the belief consistent with reality?

- How realistic is this belief?
    - Is there any evidence?
    - Where is the data that supports this belief?
- How helpful or pragmatic is this belief? Does it help me towards my goals?
    - Where will it get me?
    - Is it helping or hindering me from attaining my goals?

What is useful to remember when you dispute your irrational thoughts is that it is about challenging your belief, not you as a person. Your irrational beliefs do not define you as a person. From disputing your beliefs, the final step is the new **E**ffective belief, which is coming up with a healthier or more *rational* belief that has more helpful emotional, behavioural and cognitive consequences. One sportswoman I spoke to, Chrissie (triathlete), gave a nice illustration of how she used rational thinking in the labour process:

> *"I see a race as a microcosm of life that has highs and lows, these are not to be feared but to be embraced. We sometimes expect life to be perfect, but this is not rational." This is a really relevant example of a rational thought. It is not helpful to expect that the labour is going to be perfect, it may be a very uncomplicated birth where things go to plan, but there may still be parts of labour that are not. These are, however, not to be feared.*

You may remember from chapter 3 that I quoted from *Hamlet* – it is neither good nor bad, but our thinking makes it so. It is our interpretation of an event that influences our judgements of situations, which can influence how we feel. Feeling sad or frustrated is not always bad, and we don't need to engage in disputing our beliefs every single time we may feel a bit frustrated or upset. REBT is about helping you to gain an insight into the role that beliefs play in your response to events, especially if the event is not what you were hoping for, like a change to the birth plan. At the same time, it is important to remember that some consequences are healthy consequences, and these can result from rational beliefs. The aim is not to eradicate every negative thought that appears in your head! This is not helpful, and you'll be so tired and all consumed by this that you won't have any capacity left for anything else. If our beliefs are, however, irrational and lead to some unhealthy consequences, then it might be time to step in and dispute the irrational thoughts. If you are, on a day-to-day basis, affected by irrational beliefs and it affects your mental health, then do make sure to speak to medical professionals to help you address this.

Take-home message

1. How can self-talk help you to approach the maternity journey as a positive challenge? As an example, instructional self-talk can be useful to tell yourself what to do (approach focus), motivational self-talk can be useful to tell yourself that you can do it (self-belief) and addressing irrational thoughts can be helpful when it comes to experiencing control.

2. Don't try to focus on suppressing unhelpful thoughts. We all tend to have rather busy minds with lots of thoughts flying around, some of these more helpful than others. It is not realistic to think that you should eradicate or suppress all the unhelpful thoughts or 'silly' things you say to yourself. Suppressing thoughts in the long term takes a lot of energy. Of course, there will be times during labour when it can be useful to tell your thoughts to shut up and help you to refocus on the process, and that's okay.

3. Engage your support system to help remind you of your self-talk statements. Sometimes all you need is a little nudge to remind yourself of the self-talk, but if you have had enough, remind your support system beforehand that they don't force the statements on you either!

4. Take ownership over your self-talk statement and make sure that your self-talk statements are meaningful to you; if you feel you 'own' the statements, they are so much easier to remember when you feel under pressure.

5. Speak to someone if unhelpful thoughts get out of control. What's incredibly important is that if you suffer from detrimental self-talk, please make sure that you speak to someone about this, as reading a self-help book is unlikely to sort all of this out. A health professional, such as the midwife, might be the first point of contact, but if it starts to interfere with your daily functioning, it is important that you speak to your doctor, a registered psychologist, and/or contact a helpline such as the Samaritans. Don't be afraid to reach out, as this can also help you postnatally.

7 The power of the breath: Breathing and mindfulness-based strategies

Breathing techniques and the birthing process go hand-in-hand. Breathing techniques are popular, and have been taught for quite some time; traditionally antenatal classes would be dedicated to the art of controlled breathing through contractions. In most antenatal classes, breathing is still a key part of the curriculum. Where initially breathing techniques were taught in a set way, it is recognised that there is no need for a 'one fits all' approach. As breathing is a key ingredient for psychological strategies, such as imagery and mindfulness-based strategies, I will cover some of the basics of breathing to give you an idea of how it works, so that you can use it as part of these psychological strategies, or you can use breathing techniques on its own. In the second part of this chapter I will outline the basics of mindfulness.

What is breathing?

It feels like an odd question to ask: 'What is breathing'? as we do it all the time and it is what keeps us alive. Breathing is the inhalation and exhalation of air, where air is moved into and out of the lungs to bring in oxygen and get rid of carbon dioxide, which is a waste gas. The physiological and physical benefits of breathing during labour are well-documented, such as changes in pain threshold and reduced muscle tension. When you lose control over your breathing and find that your breathing is superficial, the effects can be rather unhelpful, the body tenses up, less blood may be flowing around your body, and you could experience weakening of lower back muscles. If we take it back to sport, when you watch a penalty shootout in football, you may notice that some football players breathe shallowly and raise their shoulders whilst breathing, instead of using a more grounded, or diaphragmatic way of breathing. Shallow breathing can influence the centre of gravity; this can affect posture and balance and as such sport performance. You may be able to imagine how this can affect penalty kicks, as well as many other sport activities. Think about kicks in taekwondo, balance beam routines in gymnastics, or a spin in figure skating. Pretty much all sport activities have a component of balance. When we consider centre of gravity, there is also a clear link with labour, where you may use squatting or are rocking back and forth on a birth ball. If your breathing strategy can make you feel grounded, then this can be an advantage. Using controlled, or intentional, breathing as a strategy is therefore an essential tool to have in your tool kit.

The brilliant thing about breathing is that it is something that we, normally, do all the time. As such, it is something that you carry with you wherever you go. Remembering that you have access to breathing as a tool is such a powerful thing, especially as it can make you feel that you are in control. Breathing is an insightful indicator of how we are doing, but at the same time you can learn to use it strategically. This is where it becomes a strategy from a psychological perspective, as engaging in controlled breathing is something that you can choose to do. Using controlled breathing as a strategy has advantages which are not only physiological (such as oxygen flow) and physical (reduced muscle tension), but also psychological. Some of the psychological advantages include pain management, it can also help reframe the way you see labour, for example, you can approach it as a positive challenge, where the task ahead feels manageable, and not a negative threat where the task ahead feels like a massive mountain that's impossible to climb. Reframing the labour as a positive challenge and feeling relaxed and calm can also help with decision-making. As we learnt from the goal-setting chapter, there are plenty of occasions when the birth plan needs to be thrown overboard and on-the-spot decisions need to be made. Using controlled breathing to get you, or remain, in a calm state can be very helpful, both for you and your birth partner.

Breathing techniques are well suited to use in combination with the other psychological strategies in your tool kit, such as imagery, self-talk, and mindfulness-based strategies; the latter I will cover later in this chapter. For example, breathing can help with how you experience pain, especially when combined with imagery. You can imagine that you are breathing in fresh oxygen to the pain and when you breathe out that with the air you breathe out the pain leaves your body. You can also combine self-talk with controlled breathing. This can be through using counting or having a breathing-related mantra that matches your breathing pattern. Perhaps something like saying 'let' when breathing in, and then 'go' when breathing out.

This is all good and well, but of course it is easier said than done, especially if you are not necessarily aware of when you lose control over your breathing; so let's have a look at some examples. If you are upset, or perhaps feel under pressure, breathing rates often speed up and you sometimes may feel you are gasping for air. Can you remember a time where you felt like this? Perhaps this was an important presentation at work, at the start line of a race, a first date, or when you had an important assessment. Spend a bit of time on reliving how that felt when your breathing pattern changed. What were the triggers? How did it feel? How did it affect your thoughts and feelings? Did you manage to get your breathing back under control? If so, how did you manage to do this?

Reflecting on times when you felt you lost control over your breathing can be insightful as an indicator to refocus and go back to the process of breathing. When you are in the middle of having lost control of your breathing and you are in pain, it can be hard to refocus. Having an awareness of what some triggers are for when you are losing control over your breathing is useful to get your focus back. Of course, the increase in oxygen that you will get to your body when you regain control over your breathing is also valuable when it comes to labour. When you are in a situation where you feel overwhelmed, do remember that there are usually people, whether at home or in the hospital, with you who can support you and remind you to reconnect with your breathing. For example, you can share any instructional self-talk to get your focus back on breathing with birth partner(s) and others who are there to support you before you go into active labour, where it can feel like it all becomes a bit much. Jo (basketball player), one of the women I interviewed for this book, had her doula remind her to use her breathing strategy, which then helped Jo to re-engage with the process. There are also various options for anaesthetics to help relieve pain, which could help if you struggle to breathe 'properly'. What is important to remember is that you do not have to rely on one single way to relieve pain, and you can draw on a combination of strategies. Having said that, controlled breathing is generally promoted as a tool in labour, and it lends itself well to be used in combination with anaesthetics in the lead-up and during C-sections. Even if you do not feel the contractions, you can still use breathing strategies for its physiological and psychological benefits, such as tuning in to the labour and feeling that you are in the present moment experiencing the birth of your child.

Here is a task you could try. Something you can do to develop awareness of how breathing works is to try various breathing rates and notice what happens, this is particularly helpful to become aware of when you are 'overbreathing', which can happen when we feel stressed. One way of becoming aware of breathing rates is through practicing different counts of breathing, where you breathe in for 6 seconds and breathe out for 6 seconds, and then reduce the inhalation or exhalation rate with 1 second. A general observation is that if your inhalation is longer than your exhalation, then you tend to feel out of breath, and as such this may be something you'd like to avoid when it comes to labour! On the other hand, a shorter inhalation followed by a longer exhalation can help to calm down. Practicing breathing rates beforehand can help you feel more confident that you can gain control over your breathing, and not let the breathing control you. Do take care to monitor your breathing when you do this task, and make sure not to push it to the point where you are getting too much out of breath. You may also notice that at different stages of your pregnancy your breathing feels different as the uterus grows. If you have any concerns about your breathing during pregnancy, please do make sure to consult with a medical professional.

Once you have established a ratio that works for you, start practicing this in a calm and peaceful place, and when you feel comfortable, you can take it to other settings. It may be that you can use it in the work-place before an important meeting, when you are doing exercise, or when you are in a busy place. There are some excellent breathing apps that you could download to your phone to help you practice. What is important is that you learn to adapt your breathing ratio, as sometimes this is needed for the intensity of a task. Imagine that you are on a training run, where the training intensity is an 8 out of 10. It can be pretty difficult to then maintain a breathing ratio of 5 seconds in and 6 seconds out! The reason I mention this is that when it comes to the transition towards the active stage of labour, contractions become stronger, the effort required intensifies, and so you may need to adapt your breathing ratio. Emma, an avid runner, whilst reflecting on what she would have done differently during labour, mentioned that she would have liked to be better prepared for the different stages of labour as she had not prepared for the pain in the early stages of labour. Having prepared how to adapt breathing strategies to the different stages of labour, not just the final stage, would have helped to ease her anxiety throughout.

A very commonly used breathing technique is diaphragmatic breathing. Diaphragmatic or 'belly' breathing is a technique that focuses on filling the lungs with oxygen in an efficient way. I often practice this type of breathing with sportspeople as it can help them to feel calmer, it can also benefit your cardiovascular responses, such as blood pressure, and hormonal changes. Simply said, diaphragmatic breathing encourages you to feel your diaphragm move when you breathe. Having your hands placed on the diaphragm (located around the base of the chest) can help you to feel the inhalations and the exhalations. With diaphragmatic breathing, you notice that your abdomen expands as you inhale and fill it with air, and as you exhale you notice your abdomen, or belly, going back in. With this type of breathing, your shoulders tend to stay still when you inhale. You can notice this by placing your hand on your upper chest, and when you engage in diaphragmatic breathing, you don't feel much movement around the chest. In essence, all the 'action' takes place around your diaphragm and belly. It's helpful to be aware that when you are pregnant the diaphragm moves up, therefore you may notice that diaphragmatic breathing may feel a bit different compared to if you have practiced this when you were not pregnant.

I would encourage you to think about situations where you can practice these breathing exercises on a regular basis, so it becomes easier to do them. Perhaps you can do breathing exercises in combination with pelvic floor exercises or when you are brushing your teeth. Maybe, when you are comfortable with the breathing exercises, you can stand on one leg (with some support if needed) and practice diaphragmatic breathing. These are just some suggestions; do what feels good for you.

By now, I hope you've gotten the idea that using breathing as a strategy has several benefits and that you can be proactive in practicing your breathing techniques. It can make a difference in how you experience pain, and it can be helpful to make you feel calmer and take you back to being in the here and now and focused on the present moment. Being focused on the present moment is an integral part of mindfulness, of which breathing is an important part. Mindful breathing is an example of this, and before I explain what mindfulness is and how can it help you in sport and during the maternity journey, I will share a brief mindful breathing exercise with you.

Mindful breathing task

Get yourself in a comfortable position and start taking slow, deep breaths. Pay attention to the air going in and out of your body, how does this feel? Feel the air fill your body as you inhale. As you exhale, your shoulders may drop and you feel the air leaving your mouth or nose. As you are breathing in and out, you may start to notice thoughts pop into your head. Whenever this happens, notice that it is a thought, and without judgement wave to the thought, as if it's a passer-by, and go back to your breathing. Breathe in, breathe out. Really notice the sensations of the breath, and the air moving around your body. If you do notice a thought distracting you from your breathing, acknowledge that the thought is there, and then gently take your attention back to the process of breathing. Breathe in, breathe out.

This exercise is not about counting breaths, it is about recognising that you have thoughts that might pop up, and without judging or analysing these thoughts, you gently move your attention back to the breath. This is quite a helpful task to practice regularly, and it is a task that is often used as a foundation for other mindfulness-based tasks.

Mindfulness: A brief overview

Mindfulness is becoming more and more embedded in sports. When we consider (high performance) sport, there is this constant evaluation of how you are doing compared to others, and factors such as avoidance behaviour, anxiety and worries, injury, unrealistic expectations, perceived pressure, and life-balance difficulties all play their part. Mindfulness can be very useful to manage these demands and move away from this constant judgement and comparison with others.

What is mindfulness? Mindfulness is 'being in the present'. It is about paying attention to the present moment, where you don't judge, you are open, accepting, and curious. You can think about it a bit like seeing the world through the eyes of a young child, as if you are experiencing the present moment for the first time. Within this, it is about observation without being critical, being kind and compassionate to yourself, and allow yourself to be where and as you are. This combination of being kind and compassionate to yourself, as well as not being critical, can be so difficult, especially in a lot of Western culture, where people are taught to be competitive, not only in sports but also in jobs, and even friendships. They often want more, do better, and a lot of people tend to compare themselves to others. Letting go off all this comparing and judging and taking on a non-judgemental focus can be hard!

A few years ago, I took a mindfulness-based cognitive therapy training course, and I remember one of the tasks vividly. We were instructed to look out of the window and focus on one scene for three minutes, with curiosity and without judgement. I remember that my view comprised a brick wall and not much more. I was a bit disappointed that I did not get to stand on the other side of the room, where there was a street view with a lot more excitement. Initially, I judged the cracks in the bricks and the unevenness of the wall. Through the exercise, I learned to observe and take in the wall for what it was, I started to notice small details and I was able to notice when my thoughts were judgemental ('Why has no one been doing anything about this wall? Why couldn't they have built that wall better or do some maintenance on it?'). When my thoughts were drifting, I learned to notice this, and gently took my attention back to observing the wall with curiosity. It was, and is, not easy, but it is now an exercise that gives me calmness. In fact, I actually found this rather useful during labour. When I was moved from the ward to the labour room, there was a screen with changing (and recurring) images. Once I was put on the oxytocin drip and the contractions started, I used this mindfulness observation task where I intently looked at one part of the image, such as the mast of a boat in the harbour, until the next image came on. For me, this was something that calmed me down and helped me to notice thoughts that were unhelpful, and to then come back to the image. Having these wall-sized big screens with images is something that is fairly new, and part of making delivery rooms more sensory, which includes being able to program the lights and have sound effects. There is some evidence to suggest that sensory delivery rooms can have a positive influence on the labour experience. Of course, not all delivery rooms have these sensory effects, and if this is something you think would be of benefit to you, you can think about ways you can mimic this, such as bringing in a scenic poster or a tablet/laptop.

As with the other psychological strategies, mindfulness is a practice. What this means is that it requires training and development over time; you can't just be more mindful from one day to the next. It is a process, and it does take time. Mindfulness is sometimes portrayed as a quick fix, but mindfulness training can be, and for a lot of people it is, hard work. The aim is not, for mindfulness or the other strategies, to be perfect at it. The aim is to learn about the different strategies, get better at them, and as such improve the psychological strategies available to you in demanding situations. Giving birth may be one of those situations!

In sport, mindfulness is often used to help reduce pressure, but mindfulness can also help with pain. Through tuning in to the pain and taking a non-judgemental approach (not 'why me, this is ridiculous, why does it hurt so much' but 'I can feel that …') the pain can become less intense. This is where something like yoga practice can be useful, to better understand your body and, in a safe environment, expose yourself to discomfort and allow yourself to tune in to how your body feels. If you are pregnant, there are some safe yoga poses that you can try this with. Especially if you have not done yoga before, ensure that you speak with your health practitioner and a qualified pregnancy yoga teacher to advise you on a pose that would work and is safe for you. When in this pose, you can use instructional self-talk to talk through a calm breathing rhythm. You can also use imagery to visualise the discomfort and imagine where the discomfort is located. When I did this with the (half) pigeon pose, I felt that this was important to ensure I would not get myself in a position that was not helpful when being pregnant! By doing this, I started to notice that the pain and discomfort actually went down, together with trying to 'just be', and not giving myself a hard time for finding this a challenging pose. I had heard and learnt about how tuning in to pain can reduce the intensity, but never actually made a concerted effort to try this. It may, of course, not work for everyone, especially when you feel overwhelmed by a wave of contractions, but it may be worth a go. As with everything, do try to practice this so that when it comes to it, you have that strategy in the 'bank' or in your toolkit on the day(s).

I do want to clarify that when I mention that you can use mindfulness as a strategy in your toolkit, that this is not necessarily the same as *being* mindful, as that is much more to mindfulness than using mindfulness strategies at select times. This is where some of the 'conflict' between the Western and Eastern approaches to mindfulness exists. Do what works for you, and if adopting some mindfulness-based strategies helps you to manage pressure and pain, then all the better. From here, we move to an approach that is gaining more and more popularity in sports, ACT, or Acceptance Commitment Therapy, which incorporates mindfulness-based components.

A big part of mindfulness is observing your thoughts, with openness and without judgement. This includes observing your thoughts before a race, training session, or maybe a midwife appointment, without labelling these thoughts as good or bad, or trying to change the thoughts. A lot of this is about 'acceptance', and this is central to Acceptance Commitment Therapy, or ACT (pronounced as the word 'act'). What makes ACT so powerful is that it focuses on accepting your thoughts and feelings as well as focusing on your values. Through a focus on acceptance and your values, the idea of ACT is to help people develop 'psychological flexibility'. In essence, it helps you to 'welcome' your thoughts and emotions, rather than fighting them. There are six principles that can help to develop this psychological flexibility; these are acceptance, values, committed action, contact with the present moment, observing self, and defusion. I will describe each of these briefly, and if you feel that you would benefit from more information about mindfulness or ACT, there are some references at the back of this book for further reading.

Acceptance is making room for sensations and feelings that are not always particularly pleasant, it is about embracing thoughts and emotions without trying to fight them or suppress the thoughts. What you try to do is to open up to these unpleasant sensations and find that they may move on, a bit like clouds in the sky. If you do not make space for the unpleasant thoughts, then they don't have the space to move on, and it's like a rain cloud being stuck above your head. It may be that, as part of your maternity journey, it is about making space for thoughts and feelings of getting a different birth experience than you had in mind rather than trying to avoid thinking about those different birthing experiences altogether. You may remember from the self-talk chapter that we have this constant chatter in our head – with acceptance, you move away from evaluating or fighting thoughts and move to observing these instead. The mindful breathing task earlier in this chapter is an example of an acceptance exercise. You can build on this mindful breathing, for example, by observing how your body feels. Scan your body from head to toe; do you feel any uncomfortable sensations? Maybe your hips ache or your back feels tight. Pick one of the sensations and really tune in to it, and observe it as if you are a stranger who has never experienced something like this before. Maybe you can give the sensation a colour, a shape, or a sound. Does the sensation move around in your body? Observing the sensations with a curiosity like this can help to distance from them, and as you start breathing into the area, you can use imagery to imagine how you can create space around the sensation. Doing so gives it space to move, and from here you can let the sensation just be. The aim is not to push it away, or to like it, but just let it be there. Of course, it might move after a while, but that is not the aim of this acceptance exercise. It is not an easy task, but it might be helpful at those stages in labour where it all feels a bit much and where it feels like the baby takes all the space!

Values is another key principle of ACT. Values are about what you want to stand for, and give us direction, and we briefly touched on values in the chapter on goal-setting (chapter 4). Values are about what is important to you; if you are clear on what your values are and feel connected to your values, then this can help when things get tough because of the direction it gives you. Knowing what you want to stand for in life and what is meaningful to you can help with psychological flexibility; you are not fighting your emotions, and you can use your values to guide and adapt to situations. This is especially helpful when you feel under pressure and don't know what to do; going back to your values can remove or reduce the pressure because it helps you to see why you might find the situation difficult. Values can be things like caring for others and the environment, patience, perseverance, kindness, hard-work, just to name a few examples of values, and they are identified by *you*, it is not about what is important to others. There may sometimes be conflicting values, and having an awareness of how your values drive your behaviour can be helpful, especially when considering committed action. Let's say that it is important for you to be physically fit. During your pregnancy, you are experiencing pelvic issues, and you cannot do any moderate physical intensity and are told to rest as much as possible for the time being. Because being active is so important to you, yet you are unable to exercise, this makes you feel cranky. You reflect on other values that are important to you, like spending time with friends and kindness, and you prioritise those values for the time being and this then gives you that psychological flexibility. Values are chosen by you; they are a guide, not an end-goal. Values are therefore not to be confused with goals, where a goal usually has a destination (getting physically stronger, improving technically or tactically and so on), values provide direction, and your goals can enable you to move in the direction you want to take. It's a bit like a lighthouse, which will keep you on track, even if you feel like you are a bit lost in stormy weather conditions.

Committed action is about taking action that is informed by your values; don't just look at the values, but 'do'. When things are getting difficult or there are too many things going on, it is easy to take shortcuts and brush aside the actions you intend to take. Perhaps you really value patience, but under pressure, you find it difficult to think clearly, and you start taking shortcuts. These shortcuts can then take you away from the road you want to be on; you can come back to the journey through committed action that is informed by your values. This could mean that you need to ask, if of course the situation allows this, for a minute or two to gather your thoughts before making decisions. It might be that you find it easier to take committed action in one setting, such as in a family or sport environment, but feel that it is a lot tougher in other settings, such as the workplace or in a medical environment. I know I talk about awareness a lot, but having an insight into which settings you find it harder to take committed action is helpful, as you can identify a setting where you might find it harder and start thinking about how you can set goals to enable you to behave in line with your values.

Present moment, or connection, is about focusing on what is going on in the here and now, and another principle of ACT. Not dwelling or ruminating on what has happened in the past or having worries about what is to come, but focusing on the moment. Perhaps you have a planned caesarean and are worried about what others may think about this decision, as in your culture, this is frowned upon a bit. Those people are not who have grown the baby inside you, you have agreed to the planned caesarean with your healthcare provider and it is your decision. Make the most out of the situation; this is your moment to meet your baby. A nice exercise to do to practice being in the moment, or connecting with the present moment, is to tune in to your surroundings and noticing all your senses. It is a bit like imagery that we spoke about earlier in the book. When you are going outside for a walk, you can stop and pause for a second and look around you, what do you see? What do you hear? What can you smell? What can you feel? Other exercises that are quite popular when it comes to being in the here and now are 'awareness of the breath' and 'awareness of the body', and there are lots of examples online on these if you do a search. When doing these exercises, you may feel that your mind gets occupied and filled with thoughts and feelings. This is completely normal, and rather than fighting these thoughts, you notice them (remember acceptance?), and go back to noticing the sensations. Practicing being in the present moment can be quite helpful to focus fully on that moment where you get to meet your baby and move away from any thoughts where you might be judging yourself! This is also a useful exercise to do when you are at the start line of a race and feeling intimidated by people around you, or after you have missed an easy shot in basketball/netball/golf and start ruminating about the miss.

Another principle of ACT is the observing self. The self is always there, and the observing self is without judgement. This sounds simple, right? Yet we are in a world where there is constant judgement, and sometimes we are our own worst critic. There is a very close link between the observing self and being in the present moment; these go hand in hand and are about being in the present. That exercise where I learned to look at the wall with curiosity was an example of when I started to engage my observing self. For once, I managed to give my busy mind, where thoughts filled with judgements were spinning around non-stop, a break. The moment, during labour, where I could let go and just focus on one contraction at a time really helped me to connect with the pain and manage it without an epidural. It was not like the pain just went away, it was very much still there, but it worked for me and it helped that I had clarity in my values and could take committed action, and I knew I had my observing self with me. For others, this may be the moment when you feel it is the right time to ask for an epidural or another method of pain relief. Whatever works best for you, in your situation, go for it. Remember that the self is there as non-judgemental observer.

Defusion is about changing your relationship with your thoughts, where in essence you are relating to your thoughts in a new way. Often, we let uncomfortable, painful, or unpleasant thoughts get to us; it's like these thoughts are merged with our self. If you can find a way to 'defuse' these thoughts from the self, they have much less of an impact. Maybe you can remember a time when you missed an easy opportunity in your sport, like an uncontested lay-up in basket-ball or a tackle in rugby, and your thoughts were similar to 'How on earth can I be such a bad player that I missed that tackle', 'I can't even make the easiest lay-up', 'I let my team down' and so on. Defusion is about taking a step back and disconnect from these thoughts. As we already noticed in the self-talk and emotions chapters, thoughts can be very real, important, clever, and also threats. Perhaps you have the thought 'I can't do this', or 'I am a failure', and it is no surprise that these thoughts can make you feel upset. Remember, thoughts are very often 'just' thoughts, and we do not need to act on each thought that we have. One way of starting to realise that thoughts are 'just thoughts' is to make yourself aware that it is a thought, by noticing that it is a thought and telling yourself (in your head or out loud) that you notice that you are having this thought: 'I am having the thought that I can't do this'. You can perhaps draw a head and write the thought down to help you step back from the thought or sing the words of the thought to a tune (maybe a way to start practicing some nursery rhymes tunes). Another way is to 'defuse' the *I*, so instead of saying 'I am a failure', you label the thinking process by stating something along the lines of 'I am a person who is having the thought that I am a failure'. It is all about taking that step back and realise that (unpleasant or uncomfortable) thoughts are just thoughts; they come and go, you can remove yourself from the thoughts, and that you do not need to let these thoughts tell you what to do.

Taken together, psychological flexibility can be very helpful to help you focus on the process and being in the present moment. Control the controllables and letting go of what you can't control is so relevant here. Having psychological flexibility and drawing on those principles such as seeing thoughts for what they are can be essential as a way to help you control those controllables, and to accept what is outside of your control to be able to let go. Both in labour and in sport, there are so many situations where you may have to deal with other people around you, such as coaches, consultants, teammates, support staff, that may trigger you to feel pressure, perhaps because different things are important to them than they are to you and your values may not align. This is not something that you can change (control) all the time, and in some situations, there is just not the scope to do so. Using the principles of ACT can help you to be more flexible and not let thoughts that are unhelpful take over.

Take-home message

1. How can breathing and mindfulness-based strategies help you to approach the maternity journey as a positive challenge? Taking committed action is an example of an approach orientation, counted and regulated breathing can give you the belief that

you can manage a one-minute-long contraction, and acceptance helps to see what is in and outside of your control.

2. Breathing is a tool you carry with you wherever you go. Because it is so readily available, we sometimes forget to tune in to it. There are so many ways you can use breathing strategically, such as to help you to calm down or you combine it with self-talk statements or imagery to help remind you to engage in diaphragmatic breathing to reap the benefits of increased blood flow and oxygen.

3. Mindfulness-based strategies can be very useful to have in your toolkit, but mindfulness tools are not the same as mindfulness. Mindfulness takes a lot of practice, and some of the mindfulness strategies covered in this chapter are just a taster.

4. Aim to approach situations with greater psychological flexibility by gaining clarity when it comes to your values. Values can give you a guide on how to act by following the light coming from a lighthouse.

5. Where in the last chapter, we focused on addressing and changing irrational beliefs, ACT focuses more on letting thoughts be thoughts and not trying to actively change them. Both approaches can be helpful tools to have in your toolbox, and it is up to you to use the tools that work for you. You may reach for one tool time and time again, and the other tool may only be used once or twice, but end up being invaluable for that particular situation.

8 Focus: Being in the moment and letting go of the uncontrollables

Focus on the moment, don't think too far ahead. You are thinking this is a contraction, and then it is over. It is the same with racing, this period of time, my leg hurts like hell, in ten km time on the run it won't, I know it, because experience tells me that. So I think that was really useful, to think stay here, stay in the moment. It is a contraction. A race will end. The baby will come out. The contractions will end. (Chrissie Wellington, former professional triathlete and Ironman Triathlon World Champion)

'I just let it happen', 'I was completely in the zone', 'Focus on the moment', these are just some examples of experiences that women have had during labour. On the other hand, quite a few women shared with me that they completely lost control over what to direct their attention to, such as 'Couldn't focus on my breathing and totally forgot what I was doing'. Of those who talked about feeling completely in the zone, some reflected on how they lost their sense of time and how things just seem to happen without them having to think too much about it. Although being in the zone where everything feels automatic and instinctive is a great feeling, it is not a necessity for peak performance, nor is it a required ingredient for a positive birth. What is useful, however, is to learn to focus in such a way that you can be in the moment and direct your attention to the task at hand. Or, when you feel you have completely lost it, that you are able to recognise this and then have a way to refocus.

Giving birth is a situation where there can be so many unfamiliar experiences, and this unfamiliarity can sometimes make it difficult to focus on the task. For example, your appearance may be a bit different from your 'normal' day-to-day appearance, you may have to poo, pee, vomit, or you might swear, shout and say things that you didn't know could come out of your mouth. If you feel self-conscious about what the midwife, consultant, or your birth partner might think, or are concerned about the impression you make on others, it can be difficult to then focus on being in the moment and direct your energy to the process of giving birth, such as your breathing technique or positioning. Of course, telling someone to not be self-conscious is so much easier said than done, some of the strategies covered earlier, such as imagery, goal-setting, and self-talk, can be useful to move your thoughts away from being overly aware of your actions and thoughts of self-consciousness, and these strategies can help you to focus on the process. This leads us to focused concentration, or focus, which will be the main emphasis of this chapter.

Focus is a word that tends to come up during birth preparation classes or during antenatal appointments. It's such a common thing to tell someone to focus, but so much harder to put into action! Imagine that you are in the middle of a contraction and suddenly the pain is so much more intense than any previous contractions, you are suddenly completely overwhelmed by the pain, and have no clue how to shift your focus to controlled breathing. At this stage, trying to be completely in the zone is not an easy task. Nor is it always advocated, as intense pain can be a warning signal to change course. Similarly, in sports, there are situations where worrying thoughts can take the focus away from being in the zone. Although you can try to tackle these worrying thoughts, this may not always be feasible in the very short term. A powerful example is Simone Biles, the American gymnast who made the decision to withdraw from two finals at the Tokyo Olympics in 2021. She explained that she had the 'twisties', which is when someone is trying to perform a skill in gymnastics, like landing a move, the body and mind are not in sync. This is a dangerous situation, which can lead to serious injuries if she were to land on her neck. Although it is unlikely that you will be doing a somersault during labour, there may be occasions where you feel a mismatch between the body and mind. At this stage, it will be helpful to recognise that this is happening and to find ways to communicate this to those around you. Developing an awareness of when you lose focus and identify ways to then refocus is a key skill in sport and will also benefit you during labour. Therefore, I will explain what focus is about and share some ideas of how you can recognise where your focus is, and how you can, if necessary, shift your focus to a more appropriate focus. This is helpful to take the pressure off, and it can also help with the decision-making process during labour and enable you to direct your attention to the controllables, rather than trying to control something that is uncontrollable in that moment. Remember that birth plan, and how it may have to be thrown overboard and you have to make difficult decisions in the heat of the moment? This is where some focusing strategies can be helpful, not only for you but also for your birth partner who may need to make decisions for you at times when you may not be able to do so.

What is focus?

We can't be focused on the 'right thing' 100% all the time, and no one is expecting this from you. What tends to differentiate sub-elite or amateur athletes from those who perform at the very highest level, is the skill to refocus when it is needed. Focus is, much like so many other psychological concepts, quite an abstract concept. So often, we are told 'come on, focus!' Sure, not a problem, but it is *what* you are supposed to focus on that makes the difference. Focus is what we pay attention to or observe. We are constantly observing something, but that might not be the most appropriate thing to focus on at that moment in time. Let's give you a sporting example:

A point guard in basketball who is known for their defensive qualities has made a couple of difficult shots in a row, and with the team only up a few points and the potential to take the leading position in their league if they win this game, the basketball player feels pressure to make more shots. They forget to do the tasks that normally make them an effective player, get frustrated after being shouted at by the coach for not 'boxing out' their opponent when rebounding, and within the timespan of a minute they make some poor decisions resulting in turnovers and three easy baskets for the other team. In this example, you can see how quickly a situation can change. This is not too dissimilar to giving birth, where you can go quickly from being completely in the zone and focus on managing your contractions to being worried that the birth is not progressing well because perhaps you are not dilated as much as you would like. Here you can see how close the link is between our thoughts (remember the chapter on self-talk) and focus. When working with sportspeople, the first step to help them focus more effectively is for them to become more aware of where their focus is. Once they have a good understanding of this, we can then put in place some tools from the mental strategy toolbox to help with the most appropriate focus. I will share two ways that I use to help with gaining this awareness, (1) attentional circles and (2) attentional styles.

Attentional circles – me and my task

When I was in my early years of training to become a sport psychologist, I worked as an assistant for a sport psychologist in the Netherlands. He shared a lot of his learning experiences and taught me about what it can be like to be a sport psychologist. One of the core aspects of his work was how to optimise focus, a tool he used with athletes were 'attentional circles', where the aim was to learn to be in the middle or center of the circle. Building on the basics of mindfulness covered in the previous chapter, I will explain what these attentional circles are about and point out how this is relevant to the labour process, especially in terms of how to get back to the task and *the zone*.

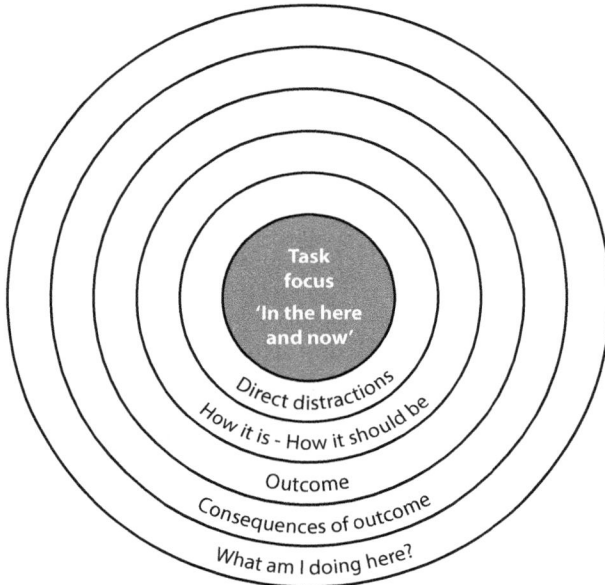

(Image inspired by Schuijers, 2018)

The middle circle is where you would ideally like to be when it comes to directing your focus. When you are in the middle circle, or circle 1, you are completely focused on the task, it is like being in the here and now. The focus is on executing the task. You could compare it to when you are colouring and are completely engrossed in filling in the lines, with a complete focus on the task at hand. But we don't always have this full task immersion, sometimes our focus drifts off and you may find yourself moving away from that middle circle. So, what might make you move away from this middle circle?

Moving away from that middle circle, you could find yourself in circle 2, having thoughts related to external distractions that are outside your control such as 'will it rain today', or 'is there going to be a large audience'? Focusing too much on these uncontrollable distractions takes the focus away from the task. Moving further away from the middle circle is circle 3, which is about comparing how it is with how it should be. Whilst the distracting thoughts in circle 2 mostly relate to the external environment, the distracting thoughts in circle 3 are more internally focused. To illustrate, a table-tennis player may focus their attention on questioning every decision they just made, and whilst they are stuck in the analysis of the last shot they forget what they need to do next, and their thoughts move away from the task. A link can be drawn with 'paralysis by analysis' or overthinking. Maybe they have thoughts like 'I should really be doing better', triggering self-doubt. In circle 4, the focus of a person's thoughts is on the outcome, such as winning or losing. These can be thoughts such as, 'Can I still win the match?', 'Is losing avoidable?', 'Am I trailing?', and the focus tends to be on the end-result, and not the task that is required at that moment in time. Thoughts around the consequences of the outcome are what circle 5 is about, and as you may have guessed by now, this is taking you further away from that focus on the task. Here, a track-and-field athlete may think about the loss of income if they don't get a qualifying time for a big event, or worry about how their support group (partners, parents, friends) respond to them performing well or poorly. The most outer circle, circle 6, has to do with thoughts around, 'What am I doing here? I can't do this', where one tends to question why they are there, and thoughts such as 'Perhaps it is better if I quit', or 'I should train more' pop up, which are not particularly helpful to focus on the here and now, and the task at hand.

How can knowing about these attentional circles help you with childbirth? If you focus too much on the outcome and uncontrollable things around you, then you lose focus on the task. This can make the labour process quite difficult. Reflecting on my experience of being told how long it would approximately take before the pushing stage would start took me away from focusing on the task of breathing through one contraction at a time. The midwife wanted to give me something to focus on, yet for me it did the opposite as it took my focus away from being in the moment and it immediately took me to the outcome (circle 4). I then needed to find energy to draw on refocusing strategies to enable me to focus again on one contraction at a time. One thing I did was redirect my thoughts back to the process, where I reminded myself that I could not rush the process, the baby is happy and will come out when they are ready, so let's go back to taking it one contraction at a time.

If you know that you are someone who is sensitive to comparing how it is with how it should be (circle 3), you can share this with your midwife, consultant or others in the room who may communicate progress with you. One of the women I interviewed, Sabine, explained how she made sure to tell the midwife not to give her any information about how long the journey might take, especially when she was giving birth to her second child. Her first child was born in three hours, and subsequent births are often (of course not always!) quicker. She did not want to think about the time frame and give herself a target time as she felt that this could only lead to disappointment if it would take longer. In essence, this is an example of circle 3 – where you draw comparisons with how it is and how you feel it should be, which takes the focus away from being in the moment. Another example of comparing how it is with how it should be was given by Pip. As a runner, she was used to racing and calculating how quick she needed to run (*need to do this pace*), and as a midwife, she was very aware of what *should* be happening at what time; it has been so many hours, so my cervix should be dilated by so many centimetres by now. She ended up clockwatching, but as you can't rush labour, this was not that helpful. Her husband (birth partner) and the midwife then decided to remove all the clocks from the room so that she could not do this clockwatching. This helped her to get her focus back on the task, and not trying to rush her way through labour. Allowing things to unfold helped her to get back to the here and now, and have that task focus.

In summary, the attentional circles can be a great visual tool to help you figure out which circle you are in and this can then act as a 'trigger' to use psychological strategies such as instructional self-talk, imagery, or breathing to help direct your focus back to the task. What the attentional circles do not specifically account for, however, is that we focus our attention in different ways. A common approach used in sports is that you can focus your attention internally or externally, as well as broad or narrow.

From attentional circles to attentional styles

Directing your attention internally means that you focus your attention inwards, such as directing your attention to the movements of the body, emotions, or thoughts. It could be imagining how you will be hitting a ball in tennis, how the racquet feels in your hand or the delight or frustration that you are feeling. Directing your attention externally has to do with focusing on something that is going on outside of you, such as an aeroplane flying over your head, wind direction or your opponent at the other side of the net. This makes sense, right? In addition to this, it is also suggested that you can have a broad and narrow focus of attention. A broad focus means that you pay attention to lots of things that are going on around you. This compares a bit to when you are approaching a crossing and you need to take in what's happening around you before you decide to cross the road. A narrow focus is when you focus on a specific point, such as where you intend to place the ball.

In essence, this means that there are four 'attentional styles', internal/narrow (prepare), internal/broad (analyse/plan), external/narrow (act) and external/broad (assess). In the figure below, I have given some examples related to sport and some to labour. You could think of some examples that are personal to you.

Example of attentional styles

External

Assess *What's going on around me? There are too many distractions, I need to change position and communicate to focus on one contraction at the time.*	Act *What do I do? Focusing on placing your feet on the floor for a stable squatting position*
Analyse/Plan *What's my plan? Let's change position, using a chair for support, and then I can focus on imaging the baby traveling down*	Prepare *How do I feel? Back is tired, feel muscle tension, chatter in mind is positive.*

Broad (left) **Narrow** (right)

Internal

So, how can you use this knowledge about these four attentional styles? Well, Robert Nideffer, a sport psychology researcher who introduced these attentional styles, suggests that we have a preferred attentional style. When we feel under pressure, we tend to go to the one that we favour. So, for example, my preferred attentional dimension is external-broad, which in some situations, is not the most useful attentional dimension. When I played basketball games and felt under pressure, one of my biggest weaknesses was that I seemed to focus so much on what was going on around me that when I was going for an uncontested lay-up, I forgot to switch to an external/narrow and internal/broad focus (for example 'hit the top right corner' and 'flick your wrist') that I had a tendency of completely mucking up the easiest of shots! Although it might feel that this is more applicable to sports like golf, football, tennis, squash and so on, it is applicable to all sports. Let's take running; if your preferred attentional dimension is internal/narrow, you may be so focused on your breathing that you may overlook that stone on a towpath causing you to trip over, or not noticing the wind conditions where you end up going too fast or getting upset about being slower than expected because of headwind. What these examples show is that we want to make sure that we do not get stuck in our preferred attentional style, as this cannot only affect performance in sports, it can also affect decision-making and our ability to take in what's going on around us. This can, sadly, also lead to injuries in sport when you don't see someone coming in for a tackle, or don't notice that the person who is cycling in front of you slows down to avoid a bump in the road.

Although this sounds very specific to sport, there is a link to giving birth. Focusing attention externally can be useful when you want to distract yourself from the pain, and this is quite a common coping mechanism that people tend to use to try to take their minds off the pain. For example, you might put on a movie to watch or chat with people to distract yourself. You might find that this distraction may be more useful when the pain levels are a bit lower. When the pain becomes very intense, sudden and sharp, it can become quite a challenge to try to use distraction techniques to move your attention away from the pain towards something else. It is also not recommended to try to continuously move your attention away from the pain, as pain may be a warning sign of the body that is important to listen to. Therefore, practicing focusing internally can be helpful. Focusing internally can help to tune in to the pain, and sometimes tuning into the pain seems to reduce the intensity (remember the mindfulness chapter). During labour, you will find that different attentional dimensions are useful at different stages of labour. For example, it can be very useful to focus inwards to imagine the baby moving down the birth canal (broad/internal) and have an internal/narrow focus when you are focusing on pushing the baby out gently and slowly. This can be quite a tough one when you need to find every bit of energy left to push, whilst at the same time trying to not push too hard! At the same time, an external focus is often needed too, especially when you need to make decisions about how to progress in labour or take in instructions from the team around you where the midwife may give you instructions to help you with pushing or holding back pushing.

To have an insight into these attentional styles, you can mimic a 'stressful' situation, such as a word-searching task under pressure (for example, by setting yourself a time limit or having someone distract you). After you finished the task, can you recall what you focused on? What were some of the thoughts you had? This might help you to give an insight as to what your preferred attentional style is under pressure. Knowing this can be useful, and you can engage your birth partner to help you shift your attention if you seem to be stuck in one of the styles and can't seem to get out of it. For example, if you are stuck in a broad/external focus and constantly tune in to everything around you, your birth partner may help you to use a self-talk statement such as 'let's tune in to the next contraction', to help shift the focus away from everything that is happening around you.

To summarise, here are two things that you can do with the knowledge of these attentional styles.

1. *Check in regularly with the attentional styles*

   In my work with runners, we have worked on identifying points in the race, or training session, where they go through the attentional styles in a way that works for them. For example, at every mile marker, they start with tuning in to their body (a quick body scan/ internal/broad) to rate their current rate of perceived effort, then they imagine running tall (internal/narrow), then they tune in to the course (weather conditions, who is running in their proximity), and then taking on an external-narrow focus, perhaps positioning in a busy field of runners. Then they do a quick evaluation of how things are going and adjust where needed. This quick check helps them to understand whether they have a bit of gas left in the tank, or whether they need to adjust their racing plan for that day. This is also important during labour as you would be a good judge of feeling what's going on in your body, but you need to allow yourself to tune in to your body and the environment. It is easy to ignore what's going on inside your body, but of course it is important to pay attention to this, and this is where regularly checking in with your attentional styles *could* be useful when you are stuck in one of the attentional styles and that style is not particularly helpful.

2. *Realise when you get stuck in one of the attentional styles*

If you notice you are getting 'stressed', and you know that there is a particular attentional style that you favour, it may be that you are sometimes getting stuck in that one attentional style. If you realise this, you can move to another attentional style. This can help with awareness and taking your focus back to what is required for the task. For example, if your favoured attention style is internal/narrow, you may be focusing so much on the pain that you become overwhelmed, taking your attention to broad/external could give you some relief, maybe some distraction from the pain, and enable you to take stock, to then plan what you will do next, perhaps focusing on your breathing strategy.

Routines

One of the things that I work on with athletes to help remind them to get back to focusing their attention on the task is to identify a routine that works for them. If they consistently and purposely engage in the routine, the chances that they get stuck in a particular attentional style or circle is less likely. Although the main purpose of routines is to help you direct your attention to the task, routines have lots of other benefits, such as feeling more confident, calm, and to help regulate anxiety. In sports, it is very common to have routines, these could be linked to a specific skill, such as particular thoughts, emotion, and behaviours one engages in just before a penalty kick in football, a 7-metre throw in handball or a serve in a racquet sport like badminton or tennis. Sportspeople also use a set routine that they engage in before the competition; this could be progressive muscular relaxation the evening before, a packing list, going through your game plan in your mind (using imagery) on the morning of the competition or a standardised warm-up with a set playlist of music. New Zealand sport teams are well-known for doing the Haka, which is a fierce ceremonial dance where the players stamp their feet, slap their body and chant loudly. Doing this before a match can help the players to get their heads in the game and get their bodies ready for action. Although I don't suggest that you go all out and do the Haka before giving birth, routines are something you could consider adding to your toolbox. The benefit of a routine is that a routine gives you something to hold on to. What is important when it comes to routines is that these are actions that you control and adapt, which makes them a bit different from superstitions, which are often built around luck and not in our control.

So how could you use routines when it comes to giving birth? As we (hopefully!) have established so far, there can be quite a few unexpected events that occur in the lead-up, and during labour. Often, we don't have control over these things, and it is unhelpful to put a lot of effort into trying to gain control over these things. On the other hand, there are a number of things that you can have control over beforehand to help you calm down, manage your anxiety, and possibly also make you feel more confident. One of those things is having the hospital bag ready to go a few weeks before your due date so that you don't have to worry about this at the last minute, researching your route to the place where you plan to give birth, and having a plan in place for different times of the day, again so you don't have to worry. It is all about controlling the controllables and letting go of the uncontrollables. As an example, my planned place for giving birth was a city centre hospital not far from a premier league football club, and I was a little bit worried about how to get to the hospital on a match day, so we researched various routes. What I had not done yet was finish packing my hospital bag; although I had a pile of stuff of what to put in it, I had not gotten around to packing, so that was a bit of a scramble when my water broke a few weeks before the due date! You can also prepare a routine that incorporates breathing, relaxation, imagery, and self-talk to help you stay calm when you maybe get a bit anxious about what's to come. You can also visit the place where you intend to give birth, if the opportunity exists, and identify a few quiet places where you could wait and do your routine. This can be quite helpful as you transition from your relaxed and calm home to a bright and busy place like a hospital setting with people around you who are unfamiliar. That having a well-practiced routine can give confidence was illustrated by Joy Black (rock climber/personal trainer) who throughout her third pregnancy, engaged herself in 'push training', where she practiced the muscles needed for pushing combined with three simple words: 'blow, hug, push'. When she was exhausted and transitioning to the pushing phase, she had this well-practiced and by now automated, routine available to her. All her mental effort went into that strategy, and whilst a lot was going on around her, she described the pushing stage as a sensory explosion; having this routine to come back to was crucial for her to maintain her focus on the task of pushing.

So how does a routine work? First, you want to identify the tasks you want to have a routine for and think about the physical and psychological aspects of that task, such as the push training example from Joy above. Also, think about what you are currently doing, does this work? Once you have established the task that you want to use the routine for, you can start 'readying'. This is where you want to move your thoughts and emotions to help you experience a positive state. Perhaps this involves motivational self-talk, or using imagery to reframe your emotional state. You also want to ready yourself physically; this could involve a tense and relax of a ligament or checking in how you are breathing. You might find that it takes a bit of practice and reflection to find which psychological strategies, such as imagery or self-talk, will work best for you to redirect an unhelpful thought or emotion to help you get into a positive state. From readying, you move on to focusing your attention, which is where those attentional dimensions come back in. For example, you can do a quick scan of the environment (external/broad), notice your thoughts (internal/broad), tune in to a specific part of your body (internal/narrow), and then focus on something straight in front of you (external/narrow), followed by doing the task. It is then, if you've got any energy left during labour, that you can evaluate how it went and make any adjustments going forward. Of course, it is helpful to practice your routine regularly in the lead-up to the task, so that it becomes second nature and is straightforward for you to use. The nice thing about routines is that you can integrate a lot of the psychological techniques that we have covered in the book.

Managing regular contractions might be a task that could be linked to a routine to help you focus your attention. For example, if you do seem to have fairly regular contractions, you can use this to your benefit. Some women have found that it was useful to integrate this with movements. In my case, as I was hooked up to a machine monitoring the baby's heart rate and the contractions, little to no movement was possible. I did use a routine where when I started to feel the contraction, I tuned in to my breathing, counted my breath and focused on the screen in front of me with moving images when I needed a distraction from the pain. Although routines are helpful and give you something to hold on to, it is okay to let go of them. If you are overwhelmed by a wave of contractions, or are moving to the next stage of labour where things may be a bit more intense, you may feel the routine is too much for you to take on, or perhaps another strategy would work better like positive affirmations or motivational self-talk.

The benefits of a routine are not just to focus your attention or to recognise that your attention is perhaps suboptimal, routines can also give you a sense of safety and security, and as such confidence that you can tackle the situation. It can also help you to learn to make associations, which during labour is especially helpful when it comes to managing the breathing to get through the pain, and you are absolutely exhausted!

Take-home message

1. How can knowing about focus help you approach the maternity journey as a positive challenge? Focusing on the process and task, and not the consequences of what may or may not happen facilitates an approach motivation. Well-practiced routines can give you a sense of belief that you know what to do next, as well as a sense of perceived control.

2. We focus on something all the time, but it may not be the thing we need to focus on at that particular moment in time. It is fine to give yourself a break from complete task focus, and be kind to yourself to acknowledge that it is pretty hard to be 100% focused on the right thing all the time. Remember ACT and psychological flexibility? That's a useful tool to have in your toolbox to help yourself with that kindness.

3. Knowing that it is normal to sometimes lose focus, what can you do to re-focus? Reflect on what your triggers are to get out of circle 1 and which tools (self-talk, imagery, breathing and so on) you can use to get yourself back into circle 1 to help you focus on the task.

4. Arousal and (physical) intensity of the task can influence your focus. Especially when the perceived effort is very high, we tend to tune in to our body. Knowing this can be helpful to understand why it can be quite difficult to focus on external stimuli. If it is important to be able to direct your focus externally, for example, to be able to take in instructions, then it is important for those around you (see also the next chapter!) to be aware of how difficult it can be to focus externally when your perceived effort levels are super high.

9 The team behind the team: Engaging your support network

Most of the chapters so far have focused on the 'individual', the woman who is giving birth, and many of the tools in the toolbox are there to help you as an individual to manage the maternity journey. This book would be incomplete if I did not cover the support team around you. The inclusion of the 'team behind the team', your own cheerleading squad, and for you to feel that you are supported, is well-needed, as a support team can be integral to bring the best out of yourself. To give you a sport example, Britta, a researcher I work with on the pain experiences of female ultra-athletes, followed two female cyclists during a two-day cycling event and one runner doing a 100-mile ultra-trail event. She interviewed them before and after the event, and any thoughts they verbalised out loud during the event were captured using a voice recorder on their wrist. When I asked Britta what she found most striking, she referred to the support network of the cyclists and the runner. Having support around them made it easier for them to do the training, and they perceived it more manageable to deal with the pain.

Overall, in sport psychology research, the overwhelming message is that perceived social support is helpful. Whether this is a rugby player who has a long-term injury preventing them from training and playing with her teammates, a runner who spends a lot of time on their training and finds it tough to juggle training with their study or work, a squash player who finds playing tournaments incredibly stressful, or a rower who is starting to feel burned out, they can all benefit from social support. It may be their coach checking in on them, friends listening to them or their family picking them up from training. Social support is not just the support team around a sportsperson, such as their coach, physiotherapist, or strength and conditioning coach, although this support team often does play a role in the sportsperson's social support system. As such, I am going to make a little side step to the support team before explaining how I see social support as a 'tool for your toolbox'.

Every sport, whether it is an individual or a team sport, tends to have some kind of support team. Depending on the level of competition, there is usually a trainer or coach and other people you train with, especially if you are part of a club or team. Sometimes the coaching takes place remotely. There may be nutritionists, psychologists, physiologists, strength and conditioning coaches, team doctors, and physiotherapists (physical therapists). Having the experience of working with a team of people around you can give you a great deal of confidence when it comes to labour, where you may need to rely on others to help you with making decisions. This is what Chrissie Wellington (triathlete) explained when I asked her about giving birth. She described it as a race, a microcosm of life, where she expected the highs and lows and embraced these. She expected birth to be uncomfortable and did not fear that. Having a team around her was important and helped her to feel in control; she verbalised this as follows:

> *Having my husband, having health care professionals in the room that I trusted was very helpful. Having a plan was important but paradoxically to be able to adapt. Knowing that other people knew about my plan. I felt a little bit more in control.*

Many women I spoke to referred to the word 'trust' in the context of the support team as an athlete. Amy Williams (skeleton) highlighted that being an athlete taught her to trust her support team and helped her to let go of the 'uncontrollables', she found this experience invaluable when she was communicating with the medical staff during labour. Thus, having experience of being part of a team and working with support staff can be really helpful. You may also have experienced, whether you were a solo/ individual sport athlete or a team sport athlete, that you did not get on with everyone in the team. That is normal and you can think about how you handled that situation at the time. What is important is, when you are part of team, to find out who it is that you can trust and feel comfortable with, so that you feel supported. In situations where the direct support team did not make you feel supported, there may have been people outside the 'sports team' such as family, partners, and friends who were invaluable to make you feel at ease. This is where social support, and especially *perceived* social support, comes in. Thus, when we think about our support team, it is not just about the ones that are directly involved, such as the coach, our team or training mates, strength and conditioning coaches, it is also important to think about family, friends, and your wider network.

Having a support network is helpful. When it comes to giving birth, sometimes you may not have a choice in selecting the support team around you, which is not surprising, considering the unpredictability of labour. You may be giving birth earlier than expected and are not able to travel to your preferred place to give birth, your midwife or consultant may not be available, the baby is in distress and you won't be able to give birth at home, you may have developed late-onset gestational diabetes, or there is the need for an emergency C-section where you have not met the team of consultants before. In these situations, you may have a fantastic consultant or midwife with whom you immediately click, or you may come across someone who you feel less comfortable with, or perhaps you feel misunderstood. This can happen. There are different reasons why you may not connect to the people around you; sometimes, it is because of a different culture, different values, miscommunication, or the urgency of the situation. Let's also not forget that if you feel stressed or are in a lot of discomfort or pain, that this can influence how you perceive others too. Paola, a Crossfit coach who works with women pre and postnatally, gave birth to her three children in the Netherlands. She is originally from Argentina, where typically women give birth in a hospital. In the Netherlands, it is relatively common to give birth at home. Although she wanted to give birth in the hospital, when she was due to have her first child and her contractions started, she was encouraged to stay at home. Because of complications, she did end up in the hospital and she was left feeling anxious and unsupported by the system after the experience. For her second and third child, she was assigned to an obstetrician in the hospital who she immediately clicked with. He offered her emotional support, and he was able to help her with settling her anxiety. She was feeling supported and found this very helpful when going into labour with her second and third child.

As Paola's example illustrates, to be able to (emotionally) connect with the midwife or the obstetrician can be incredibly helpful. If you feel that, for whatever reason, you don't have an emotional connection, remember that it is probably not reasonable to expect that you click with every single person you meet, and that is okay. You may still have access to emotional and social support from your (birth)partner, family, doula, or a friend. Feeling supported can make women feel more confident during labour and benefit their emotional state. It may be that the support is not always face-to-face, but you can still feel supported remotely. It can also be helpful to start thinking about ways that you feel supported when the occasion prevents you from having your preferred (social) support team physically there. Of course, the pandemic has made us so much more aware of how important it is to have access to this social support, but let's not forget that before the pandemic, women had to give birth without their preferred social support network present, and it will continue to happen in the future. For example, you can think about those who give birth in a different country to their family or whose partner may be deployed abroad on an assignment. Nevertheless, having social support is so important and we need to keep emphasising this, as it can make you feel calm and less anxious about what's to come, even if the support is not physical and in person.

Let's take a little step back and outline what different types of social support there are, as this can help you to identify what support can do for you. Some types of social support are more about providing physical help and service, such as helping you lift something heavy, doing the housework, cooking you a meal, lending you maternity clothes, or offering you transport, such as a lift to an appointment. Support can also be about providing advice, suggestions, and information. Medical staff in the hospital might explain the different stages of labour to you during a midwife appointment; they may give you leaflets or signpost you to websites with useful information. This informational support can be helpful, and there are plenty of women who feel supported by the information that is offered to them. Informational support is, however, quite different from emotional support, which is about showing care, empathy, and trust. An antenatal class teacher might give you the contact details of a support group for parents who have had difficulties conceiving after you shared with the teacher how anxious you are about being pregnant and giving birth after having tried to get pregnant for a very long time. In another situation, someone might give you a general leaflet that is irrelevant, or even inconsiderate, considering your situation, and as such you may feel that you are not being listened to or cared for. In situations like these, you may feel unsupported. It can be hugely challenging to deal with difficult and unexpected situations, you just can't always deal with things all by yourself and it's helpful to, if possible, actively seek out support that is emotional, informational, and practical. Sometimes, social support is a combination of these. When Funmi, a personal trainer, was exhausted during her very long marathon labour and found it mentally hard ('I can't do it'), the midwife used positive verbal encouragement, 'You've been doing it!' and non-verbal encouragement to give Funmi the self-belief that she was doing well and that she had been pushing for all this time. This was helpful, because as she had an epidural, she felt unsure about whether she had been pushing, and as such it also served as informational support. Together with her husband's encouragement and the information that he could see that the head was coming, she was re-energised to push her baby out.

It is so important that it is not just the *objective and received* support that is considered, but the perceived support as well. The objective support can be relatively easy to identify, such as the information you have received from the midwife, the sharing of the household chores, or someone driving you to appointments. Your birth partner may come to all your appointments, but may not really know what to do when the labour starts and therefore although they are there in person, you may not perceive it as support. Or you feel completely confident that your partner knows exactly what you need, and you feel completely supported, like the example of Funmi above.

Sometimes you may not feel supported initially, perhaps because of communication difficulties, cultural differences, or the stress you perceive. To give you an example, shortly after I was moved to the labour room, a group of medical staff entered the room and outlined the next steps. Information was offered; yet I felt that I was not given a voice and did not perceive them to be supportive. Despite wanting to have an active labour, I had a ton of wires around me that were not very long, and as such I ended up battling through the contractions lying on my back and I felt misunderstood by not being offered alternatives. Although I felt unsupported at this stage, this changed throughout the labour when I build an almost silent relationship with the midwife; I felt she was there for me, and she helped me to relax. This was very helpful when focusing on the final stages, and I started to feel that she was there with me on my journey to unconditionally support me. Together with the senior midwife she was fantastic in those final moments, and I am so pleased that I did not let my initial frustration take over the experience. Thus, perceived social support can evolve and grow over time, perhaps a bit like a relationship.

Reflecting on my personal situation, there may have been some cultural differences; I grew up in the Netherlands at a time when it was common to give birth at home (I was born at home) without medical pain relief. Despite having lived in England for many years, at times I still experience a culture clash when it comes to communication, especially under stress. Me having had to abandon my birth plan, feeling upset about this, and trying to shift my mindset on to a different birthing experience took a bit of mental energy, and together with my rather task-oriented mindset, there was a mismatch in expectations and being able to connect emotionally with those in the room. This can happen, and therefore it is helpful to remind yourself that those around you have the best interest of the baby and you at heart. The word 'midwife' means 'with-woman'. They are there with you, on your journey. What would have really helped me and my birth partner to make decisions and perceive more support and empowerment from the start, is the BRAIN acronym. What would be **B**enefits of this option, what are the **R**isks, what are the **A**lternatives, what does your **I**nstinct tell you, what happens if you do **N**othing. It gives you that opportunity for a dialogue with the midwife or consultant, and clarify some of the questions you may have. This is helpful as it can result in making you feel more part of what is happening.

Many aspects can influence a potential mismatch between received support and perceived support. There are cultural differences, especially in big multicultural cities like London, but also aspects such as how you believe pain should be managed and so on. This is no different in sports. In some sports, the culture might be to push through the pain and to not share that you are not feeling well, or that you are having an injury. Therefore, it is important to identify if there are any support mechanisms that you can turn to and realise that you often can't control how the support staff offers you support, or how you perceive this support. But overall, remember that it is not about the quantity of social support, in the end it is about the quality, and that you feel that you are supported.

How to engage your support network? What are strategies that you can use?

Knowing that support can come in many different shapes and forms is helpful to develop awareness of which sources of support you may have in place and which ones you may need to seek out more. Have a look at the list below for some examples of the different sources of support and make a list of which ones you have in place and feel are helpful to you, maybe also the ones that are less helpful to you, and the sources of support that you feel you could develop and strengthen.

Examples of support

Books	Online forums	Social media	Friends
Midwife	WhatsApp group	Birth class	Leaflets
Family	Research Articles	Doula	Family doctor/GP
Birth partner	Telephone helplines	Physiotherapist/ physical trainer	Spouse/Partner
Antenatal class teacher	Blogs	Work colleagues	Sport teammates

I will give some examples of situations where you can think a bit outside of the box in terms of support. Firstly, let's talk about the primal nature of giving birth and how this can affect the support network around you. Giving birth can be pretty primal, with lots of blood and mucus. While some women feel incredibly powerful, the lead-up to giving birth may be one of those moments where you feel vulnerable or exposed. When I recall my experiences, it was a situation where I just had to let go of any feelings of embarrassment and I had to tell myself that midwives have seen it all. In these moments of vulnerability, it is important to feel that people do not judge you so that you can completely focus on the labour. If you need to pee, do it! Although instrumental and informational support where help, advice, and information are provided is important, this emotional support, where you feel cared for and where you can let go of feelings of embarrassment, is integral to the birthing experience and this can contribute to a beneficial hormonal state. Remember, those physiological and psychological experiences go hand in hand. Without a doubt, midwives and consultants have experienced it all and do not care what you look like, that you are stark naked, or how loud you shout. If this is something you know you're going to find difficult, do share this angst with your midwife and with mothers who have recently given birth, as they can share their experiences with you and reassure you that these experiences are normal.

This primal experience may be something that your (birth) partner is not prepared for. They may have no idea how you will respond when you are in intense pain or discomfort, especially if they have never seen you suffer. It is also really difficult to expect them to put overboard all their feelings when they see the person they love and care for in pain, vomiting, or haemorrhaging. As such, do consider how you can prepare your birth partner for these situations. For example, antenatal classes can be very useful in the preparation for your (birth) partner to attend. Furthermore, can you recall any situations where you experienced intense discomfort or pain, perhaps a sport injury? How did you respond? Was your birth partner, or someone else close to you there? What was it about their support that you felt was useful and what was perhaps not so useful? Those are all considerations that can help your birth partner prepare for those situations. They may also want to watch, if they can bear it, different labour situations so that they don't feel thrown into the deep end, or speak with a friend who has recently been a birth partner, to understand what it can be like to be there at a birth. Emma, a runner, ran a marathon and trained for marathons with her husband, and he had seen her in situations where she felt anxious and wanted to give up. Knowing that he has seen and supported her during her highs and lows, led her to completely trust him and this gave her the confidence that he would stay calm when she'd be anxious and in a vulnerable state during labour.

The previous task was about thinking about sources of support. Now think about these sources more practically. Who can you turn to? The following task is about identifying who is in your support network, whilst drawing on the different types of support (emotional, instrumental, informational). Some of these sources of support may not be present during labour, but you could communicate with a friend or family member, send them messages, call them, and so on. Do make sure that you manage expectations, and that you don't feel obliged to send replies to their messages when you are in the middle of labour or immediately after giving birth! If you see some gaps in types of support, you can start thinking about ways you could increase your support system. Perhaps you could benefit from some more informational support by joining an antenatal class or an online support group. Or perhaps you are more in need of cultural support if you are giving birth in a different country or culture, and you can search for details of support groups. Of course, this is not always possible, and you may find it very difficult to approach new people and seek out support. Online support forums can be useful, yet do make sure that for medical advice, you rely on people with medical expertise and appropriate qualifications.

As a task, you can write a list of the different people who are in your support system. You can think about the antenatal groups or pregnancy exercise classes that you may be part of, a group chat and so on. If you know any other women who have recently given birth or are about to give birth, you can ask them to write a list as well and compare notes. You may just turn to one or two people, and as you do not always know how you respond in a demanding situation like giving birth, it may well be that you end up finding perceived support from an unexpected source and therefore it is good to be open to receiving support from people who you may not have thought you'd turn to. Remember that although information is a useful resource, pay attention to where you get your information from. That is, you want to make sure to find a balance in where you get your information from, don't just rely on 'Dr Google', or social media. You want to check the credentials of those offering the information, what is their professional background? When it comes to statistics, don't only look for relative risk (such as 'twice as much'), but also absolute risk (what are the actual numbers) as well as the context (who do these numbers apply to). I would also encourage you to speak to a few women who have positive birth stories to share, so that you can feel empowered.

Turning available and received support into perceived support

Now you have started to think about your support network, you can focus on how to make best use of these. You can also consider how you can turn some of the available and 'received' support into 'perceived support' to help you feel more confident that you have people and organisations to support you. The first step is to engage in a conversation to clarify your needs with your support network. Think about who is important to you and write down what you need from them in the different phases of the lead-up and during labour. You may think that they know what you need, but there may well be a bit of a mismatch between what your support system thinks you need and what you feel you need. Having a conversation about this beforehand will be useful. As such, go back to the different types of support you identified earlier, focus on the key people there, and reduce the gap between their and your expectations. You may find it useful to use your birth plan if you have one as a basis of some of these conversations and discuss what the alternative options are. Having thought about and discussed the alternatives beforehand can make it a lot less stressful when things are not going to plan. Remember if-then planning from chapter 4? This is a time when you could implement an if-then plan.

Clarifying what you need from your support network and reflecting on how you may act differently under pressure compared to those in your support network is a good exercise, because, although social support is 'supposed' to be helpful, some research does suggest that the story is a little bit more complicated than 'social support is always helpful'. For example, there are many individual differences, to illustrate, you have a tendency to use avoidance-type strategies when in pain, but your birth partner is someone who has a 'let's get on with it' approach. This difference can cause pressure and perhaps even arguments, when really what you need is a calm and relaxed environment. Therefore, it is important to consider these individual differences, and it is helpful to cover how you normally tend to cope with difficult situations in your conversations with your support system. If you know that your default option is to be nervous and anxious, then it is helpful to make your support network aware of this and discuss how they can best help you in potentially stressful situations. Similarly, if you tend to stick your head in the sand under stress, try to make your support network aware of this, as it may mean that you could benefit from help with decision-making or a 'wake-up call' when you feel stuck. An example of using your support system to help you when you feel a bit stuck was given by Funmi; her husband drew on her experiences with high-intensity interval training (HIIT) when she found it difficult to catch her breath in between contractions. He reminded her how a contraction could be like a HIIT session where you can catch your breath in between the intervals. She felt that this was helpful as it drew on something (HIIT) that was meaningful to her and that she knew she had done success-fully (recovery in between tough intervals) before.

It is important to remember that you don't always know how you will respond in a situation like giving birth, and although you may have thought that you would like to have your feet massaged, you get irritated when your birth partner attempts to do so. Or you were adamant that you did not want an epidural, but actually you prefer to have one. It can be very confusing for a birth partner when you change tune, but at the same time, it is important for them to understand that this is quite common and for you to have these conversations with them beforehand. Communication is key! All sorts of swear words may be thrown at the birth partner, again it's important to not take this personal as a birth partner. According to Pip (midwife, runner, mum), what's really key is that the birth partner is present and observant, and ready to step in when support is needed. This can be practical, such as the birth partner being in charge of food and drink, making sure that you are hydrated and properly fuelled, checking in if you need to empty your bladder, and help to support you to change position and having a good understanding of what these physical birthing positions are. They can also help to check if you need reminders to use psycho-logical strategies, for example, a birth partner could notice when your shoulders start to tense up or you tense your jaws. This may be a trigger for them to help remind you to focus on your breathing, or to do a tense and relax. Generally, the consensus from the research and the field seems to be that when a woman in labour experiences that her feelings are understood and that they are supported by someone like their partner, the midwife, a doula, friend, or family member, they tend to have a better experience. As such, if you can, make sure that you clarify your needs with your support network, and have an open conversation on how you manage stressful situations and deal with pain.

There may be also difficult conversations to have with your support network. Perhaps you are very close to your mother or sister, but prefer to not have them involved when you are giving birth. You are aware that she would love to be there for you, and you feel that she will get upset when you tell her that you don't want her to be physically there. This can be a tough conversation, yet important to tackle well before the due date to avoid this lingering on your mind. You could practice difficult conversations with someone close to you to help you feel more confident going into the conversation. One of the women I spoke to had separated from her partner and felt it would be too difficult to have him present during labour. In addition to preparing having this difficult conversation with him and talking about ways how he could be involved in the birth, such as cutting the cord, she also spent time identifying how she could ensure to have a support network that would work for her. Friends had offered to be her birth partner, but as this was her second child, she was aware of how unpredictable labour can be and she knew that friends may not be available at that particular moment. Having learned more about the birthing process, she decided to hire a doula to help give her the confidence that there was someone with her who would give her informational, instrumental, and emotional support, such as reminding her to engage with her breathing, and the doula could help make decisions. Once she was in the early stages of labour, she sent messages to those who she wanted to be part of the birth, which was also a way of reaching out for support.

Take-home message

For your birth partner and others in your support network:

1. In the lead-up to birth, spend some time to think about what your partner needs. Also check in with your partner what words of encouragement they find helpful. These don't have to be long sentences, but short and powerful statements such as 'I am here for you' and 'I love you' can be empowering. There is a lot of power in what you say and positive reinforcements are incredibly empowering.

2. Know what's in the birth plan, and discuss what alternative options there are well before labour starts. This means that if Plan A is not on the cards, you already know what Plan B and C could look like, and you can help your partner make sense of this.

3. Reflect beforehand on how you, as a birth partner, can cope with seeing someone you love or care for being in pain or discomfort. Educating yourself about the labour process can be really empowering and helping you to accept this. Having thought about this beforehand may help you to feel less overwhelmed so that you can be there to support your partner.

4. During birth (i): Stay respectful and non-judgemental throughout, and try to refrain from asking too many questions. A question like 'how are you feeling?' can hit the wrong note if your partner is suffering and trying to focus on managing a wave of intense contractions. If your partner wants to share how she feels, she will (hopefully!) make sure to tell you. Labour takes such a humongous amount of effort that a woman does not necessarily have the energy to answer your questions, and this is completely normal. Avoid inappropriate jokes or derogatory comments at all costs, as these can have a long-lasting (negative) effect.

5. During birth (ii): Don't be disheartened when a woman who is giving birth shouts and swears. This is normal, and sometimes it may be better to just be there for her, whether that is by holding her hand, breathe with her, or making sure you give her sips of

water. It can be tough to be in a situation where you want to do something to help, but feel helpless as you can't take away the pain. Sometimes less can be more, it is not about you, and this is not the time to make it about you. One mother summarised it as follows: Just be there for me and be prepared to have very little rest.

For you:

1. Invest in your support network when you are ready. We know that a broad support network is helpful, and investing in this whilst you are pregnant can be helpful during the post-partum period too.
2. If there are any difficult conversations with people in your support network, such as family members, make sure that you tackle these early on so that it does not keep lingering on in your mind and you can focus on getting ready for the birth.
3. Communicate your needs with your birth partner and spend some time checking for each other's understanding of these.

10 Bringing it home: The post-partum period

And there you are, ready to welcome the little one to the world!

The focus of this book up to this point has been on how you can learn from sport psychology in the lead-up to and during childbirth; we considered how you can draw on your experiences from playing sports to help understand how you may have already been using sport psychology strategies, and reflected on how these strategies can translate to giving birth. Once the baby has arrived, there is the birth of the placenta, the health checks, and of course the post-partum period where you adjust to a new life and a new you. How can you use some of the knowledge in this book during this period? Also, what can you take away from your maternity journey? Taking the time to reflect on your birth story may not be the first thing on your mind when adapting to the changes happening in the post-partum period. When you are ready, decompressing your emotions and feelings, as well as reflecting on your experiences, can not only help you to put your labour and maternity journey in perspective, moreover it can allow you to gain insight into what you have achieved. We will get to this a bit later in this chapter; first, we will focus on what's happening in the post-partum period and how you could use some of the psychological strategies we covered in this book.

Let's turn to the post-partum period. Once the baby has arrived, the so-called 'fourth trimester' starts, which is when you adapt to a new life with a baby, and it is also the time that the baby adapts to life outside of your womb. If this is your first baby, remember that it is also the birth of a new mother, and with this comes a change to your identity and how you see yourself. It takes time to develop and embrace this new sense of self. So much is changing, and then there is this little person who is completely relying on you. With all these changes, the post-partum period can be very much a rollercoaster, physically, hormonally, and emotionally. It can be so hard to make sense of this rollercoaster. Some days you feel great and on top of the world, while the next day you may feel deflated, perhaps because your body does not feel quite as strong as you were hoping for, or you are hungry, tired, and physically exhausted. Then there are also the 'baby blues', most likely caused by the drop in hormones after giving birth.

Baby blues and post-partum depression

Most women do experience some baby blues, which could involve crying, feeling that it's all a bit much, not quite sure what to do, and feeling fatigued. The baby blues usually last for two weeks or so. Knowing that this is normal can be helpful, as you don't feel the need to fight this. Moreover, you can mentally prepare yourself that this is likely to happen, and you can draw on your social support network to help you during the baby blues. At this stage, it is also important to point out that baby blues are not the same as post-partum depression, whilst baby blues may ease off after two weeks and your mood states are generally positive, post-partum depression is a serious condition that requires help. Some symptoms of post-partum depression, as specified by the National Health Services (NHS) in the United Kingdom, are feeling down, not being able to feel happy, feeling you are worthless, finding it difficult to concentrate, struggling to leave the house, withdrawal from others, issues with sleeping, finding it hard to look after yourself and the baby, and alarming thoughts. The NHS suggests that around 1 out of every 10 women is affected by post-partum depression in the year after the baby is born, and partners and fathers can experience post-partum depression too. It can sometimes be difficult to distinguish between baby blues and post-partum depression. Therefore it is important to speak to your healthcare provider if you have any concerns whatsoever.

Adapting to a new life and a new you

The post-partum period is for you to adapt to a new life, a new you. This period may not only be physically challenging, your body has gone through some radical changes, from growing a person inside you to delivering this baby into the world, there is the change in hormones, and it can be mentally challenging too. It is important to allow yourself time to adjust to all of these changes and to take it one day at a time. It's a bit like the task focus we talked about in chapter 8. Yet, focusing on taking it easy can be difficult. You may feel you are being pulled in different directions by your own thoughts and the external environment. Maybe you feel pressure because you are worried about what others think (circle 2), you compare yourself to who you were before giving birth (circle 3), or aspiring to be back to what you were before you were pregnant straight away (circle 4). Giving birth is, however, not a competition, and the post-partum recovery is not a race. As such, these comparisons are not helpful. Especially during the first few months after giving birth, the focus could be on embracing kindness and showing compassion to yourself. My advice is also to focus on your individual journey and try to avoid questioning too much about why your journey may not look the same as others as comparisons to others could be another source of pressure placed on yourself. When you consider the drop in hormones, there are massive differences how female bodies respond to this, and really there is no point comparing yourself to others as there is no such thing as two people having a completely identical body. Having said this, as you are entering a new phase of your life, having doubts is normal. Going on your own journey and 'getting rid' of having too many expectations takes, as Chemmy Alcott (alpine skiing) explained, a huge amount of confidence, without feeling the constant pressure of what others do and debating whether what you do is the right thing. She also explained that through the ups and downs and all the injuries she had encountered in her skiing career that she felt that she was capable of riding the post-partum rollercoaster. To help you notice that you are holding those comparison thoughts, you may find it useful to, at regular intervals, take yourself back to the attentional circles (chapter 8) and notice where you are with your thoughts. If it is a day where you feel frustrated, it can help to notice this frustration. Noticing that you feel frustrated can then act as a reminder that you are in that comparison mode, and help you to let go of the frustration.

Going back to the post-partum period and adapting to a new life, having a human growing inside you will have a major impact on your body. This impact can be experienced in so many different ways, and is not to be underestimated. Some women are able to walk immediately after giving birth, some won't, and for others the birth experience made them feel like 'superwoman'. I also spoke to women who explained that they were taken aback by how long they felt pain and discomfort after giving birth, and that they were not prepared for this pain afterwards. Even with similar types of birth experiences, the impact on the body varies. This is a bit like a sports injury, such as a torn knee ligament, where you may be given an average recovery time. But an average is just that: an average. So many factors can influence this recovery time, and not all of these are within your control. Some sports people try to beat the recovery time given to them and forget to listen to their body. This is no different when it comes to the post-partum period. You may be someone who is very competitive and when you are playing sports constantly wanting to beat others, or when you see someone ahead of you, that you want to race them. This can be helpful in competition and to give you that initial drive to find energy to push yourself, but when returning from giving birth, or returning from a sports injury, wanting to be better than others is not always that helpful. You need to listen to your body (and mind!) to understand when it is ready to return to action. Even though a doctor tells you that you are 'good to go' after your six/eight-week check, do you know what 'good to go' actually means? What are the types of things that *your* body could do at this stage? Also, are you mentally ready? If you find this difficult, perhaps because you have always pushed through injuries or pain, then it is definitely worth seeing someone like a women's health specialist to make sure that you understand what your body can do.

It's also worth remembering that when you train for an event like a marathon or start pre-season training for football, you tend to build up your mileage or strength gradually. Reminding yourself of this can help to get yourself mentally ready and alleviate those doubts you may be having, perhaps because you feel your body is not as strong as you hoped. This is quite normal, because although your body may look ready from the outside, you don't necessarily know if it's ready on the inside. It is important to strengthen the necessary muscles before moving on to higher-intensity exercise because what is not always known is that you can do more harm than good by returning to intense physical activity too quickly after giving birth. The type of exercises that are suggested to start off with may also be quite different from your pre-pregnancy workout routine. As Joy, a personal trainer working with women post-partum, explained, you need to train the body and mind how to train again. Tuning in to the improvements you are making whilst strengthening muscles can boost your self-belief and remind you of those times when you were making progress when learning a new skill, or doing a different type of workout.

With all the changes and demands you might be experiencing during the post-partum period, physically as well as mentally, this is the time to come back to some of the psychological strategies covered earlier in the book. I already briefly mentioned how you could use the attentional circles to help you become aware of comparison thoughts that you might be holding. What are other strategies you could draw on to help you in the post-partum period? I will give a few examples of using goal-setting, if-then planning, and self-talk.

It's your own race at your own pace

Goal-setting can be very helpful to help with pacing. You may aim to get back to where you were before you were pregnant, but that is not always realistic, especially not in the period straight after giving birth (the fourth trimester). Of course, there are professional athletes who are back to playing competitively within months; let's remember that there is often an entire support system around them that ensures that they are ready for a safe return to sport. Even if you are a professional athlete or relying on your income from sport and exercise, there are so many factors influencing the return to sport that it is helpful to consider this as 'running your own race and going at your own pace'. If you have planned for the post-partum period beforehand and have an adaptable pacing strategy, it makes it easier to manage those days when you feel tired and perhaps feel upset about not being ready to return to full action yet. Thus, you can use pacing as a tool to slow down or speed up based on an assessment of how you feel on that day, not based on a pre-set plan that does not take into consideration your individual progress. At the same time, recovering from giving birth is not the time to 'wing' your workout plan and you want to make sure that you have a plan in place that focuses on recovering from giving birth.

Useful to combine with pacing, an if-then plan can remind you to take it easier on the days when it's tough and your body and mind need rest. For example, you have signed up for a (post-partum) exercise class with a friend and arranged it at a time when someone helps you with your baby, but your breasts are aching, you feel grumpy, whilst at the same time you are putting pressure on yourself that you *must* go to the exercise class and not let your friend down. If this happens, what can you do to manage that situation and do it in a way that you look after yourself and you don't feel guilty about letting your friend down or feeling bad about not doing the exercise class? This action will form the 'then' of your if-then plan. Having thought about this beforehand can prevent the feelings of guilt and it can kick into action your plan to manage the situation. Perhaps your if-then plan is, 'If I feel like crap and have signed up for an exercise class with a friend, then I will remind myself that I am recovering from giving birth and that it is okay to not feel up for the class and stay at home or go for a walk instead'. As you may recall from chapter 4, if-then plans can be helpful because you will have already thought about ways to deal with the 'if', and as such you may feel more confident that you can manage the 'if', or you don't feel so overwhelmed by having to think about a way to deal with the 'if' in the heat of the moment. So much focus is on pregnancy and labour, and then on the baby, that sometimes 'critical situations', or 'ifs' *you* might experience during the post-partum period are not considered. Therefore, this may be a good opportunity to speak with some women who have recently given birth to ask about some of the struggles they have encountered and how they managed these. Of course, everyone's journey is different, yet there may be some commonalities that you can learn from.

Goal-setting can also be a helpful strategy to keep you focused on your own journey and focus on the process, not the outcome. Setting yourself goals can be helpful to get you out of the door, but do make sure that you are honest with yourself in terms of what you can and cannot do. The speed you may have been able to run before you got pregnant, how high you could jump, how much weight you could lift, or how strong your core is, it will take some time to pick up. When I was cleared to do higher-intensity exercise again, I was so excited to go out for a jog, yet I made myself a promise to take it easy and stop halfway for a stretch, and leave any type of running watch at home. This was so helpful, as I normally get carried away. I was only away for 20 or 30 minutes, but it was one of the first times I went outside by myself; I just really enjoyed being outside, just me, for that time. Following on from that first jog, I had set myself a few goals and was looking forward to getting back to strength to start playing more high-intensity sport and running at faster speeds, as well as joining workout groups where I could take my daughter to. Unfortunately, the pandemic and subsequent lockdowns started not long after. I adjusted my goals and focused on doing activities that were manageable within an apartment. It did take a bit of an adjustment; having set myself those goals for home workouts helped me to have a purpose beyond the day-to-day life of living in lockdown.

Goals can be very helpful in giving you a purpose, but at the same time, it is important to be flexible. Feeling that you have to achieve a goal can add a lot of pressure, and not having any flexibility in your goals can add to the pressure. It is okay to adapt goals, especially when your life conditions have changed. As you are adjusting to a new life, it is helpful to give yourself that permission to work around you and the baby and adapting the goals you may have set for that day. It is helpful to remember that on top of everything, especially if this is your first baby, it is not just the birth of baby, but the birth of a mother too. Although there is a lot of focus on the birth and on the baby, it is important to acknowledge that your identity, the way you see yourself, is likely going to change. For most, having a child is a big life transition. It's not only about how to adapt your daily life and routine, for many women it is also a big change to what's important for you and how you see yourself. Maybe you don't see yourself predominately as an athlete, exerciser, career woman, you name it, anymore, but you are now trying to slot in the role of being a mother too. This new identity can influence goals you are setting. Doing this in a way where you set goals that you are passionate about yet are feasible for this 'new identity' will be helpful to reduce pressure you could put on yourself otherwise. Navigating this new sense of self and 'developing' a new identity can take some time, and can be confusing at times, and that is okay. After all, you did not develop your 'pre-mother identity' in a few months either!

Remember that rest and recovery can be incorporated into your goals too. Your boundaries of what you can do may have also changed, which could be the result of the changing perception and awareness of what your body is capable of. In her research with elite athletes returning to sport after giving birth, Kelly Massey noted that one of her participants focused on their 'post-baby personal best', which is a great example of taking into consideration the new life conditions. Changes in perspective and having multiple hats might make you appreciate and re-find the love and passion for your sport, which can inform the goals you set too. Doing your sport and exercise because you enjoy doing it can make it so much easier to get out of the door because it is something that *you* want to do. Linked to this, in addition to the strategies I recapped above, gratitude is something you may be able to draw on too. A goal could be to once a day ask yourself the question, 'What is one thing that I am grateful for today?'. Doing this can promote you being compassionate to yourself which can be a really useful way to reduce negative emotions and 'self-criticism', and you can draw on some of the strategies we covered in the book to help you with this such as acceptance, breathing, imagery, and self-talk.

Speaking of self-talk, a nice illustration of how self-talk can be used in the post-partum period was given by Amy Williams. She shared how painful she experienced breastfeeding to be, especially at the start with the milk coming in, her boobs being rock-hard, and experiencing mastitis. She used self-talk, reminding herself that 'it is just a phase', and 'you're going to get through this', over and over again. She also recalled using her social support network, having a video call with one of her close friends (a free diver), who gave her an 'athlete' pep talk. She told Amy she'd get through it, it will get better, to 'dig deep', and that she could do it. She felt that this verbal encouragement and reminder that it was temporary and that the pain would go away helped to give her the confidence that she could manage the situation.

This is also a good time to revisit your social support network and re-emphasise how useful it can be to draw on social support as a strategy. Chemmy Alcott explained that when she was an athlete, she thought that she could do everything, but she learned that she needed to adjust expectations after having her first baby and that she needed to ask for help. For example, breastfeeding was tough, but being an athlete taught her the importance of reaching out, and as a result, she found support groups that helped her on her breast-feeding journey. The point here is that it is important to make roles for the people around you, don't try to do it all yourself. Although you may not come from an elite athlete background where you've had a support team (coach, physical therapist/physiotherapist, sport psychologist, nutritionist, strength and conditioning coach, lifestyle coach), that does not mean you can't build a support team around you. Friends can be your nutritional support by making you some meals, or perhaps sign you up for a meal plan to ensure that you get some healthy and nutritious food in you (so important when you are sleep-deprived and recovering from labour). Family or friends can be your 'kit manager' and help with cleaning and tidying up. Your partner can be your coach, making sure to help you stay grounded and not comparing yourself to everyone else around you. Your ante-natal group or siblings can be your teammate, and then there are also plenty of postnatal exercise or yoga groups to help you get back to physical activity in a responsible manner, without rushing it too much. Ultimately it is about you creating a support network that works for you, and having thought about this before giving birth is important. You may need a bit of time before letting in the different people of your support network, these support networks may be there at different steps along the way, or the people in the support network need some time to learn how to fit with your new life, and changed identity, and that's okay. It is your journey, and you are finding your way.

Navigating the emotional rollercoaster through decompression

Let's come back to that rollercoaster of emotions. Many women experience intense emotions after giving birth. This is no surprise, as it is a major event and it can take some time to (emotionally) recover from this. Although it can be tempting to suppress or push away some of those intense emotions, this can be rather unhelpful as it costs a lot of energy and often the intense emotions will find their way back. One approach that may be helpful to make sense of your experiences and emotions, and help you to enjoy the post-partum period in a healthy way is through decompression. Going back to sports, there are major events, such as the Olympic Games, where athletes experience intense emotional rollercoasters. To help recover emotionally from a major event, the English Institute of Sport developed a structured debrief process with the aim to process the emotional rollercoaster of major events. There are four stages to this (1) hot debrief, (2) time zero, (3) process the emotion, and (4) performance debrief. We will focus on the first three stages here.

The hot debrief is the time immediately after the event, with the intention to offload any thoughts and emotions that come to mind. This can be a 'muddle' of thoughts, feelings, and sensations. It can be those text messages that you send to friends in the immediate aftermath, a chat with your partner, a voice note to yourself, or some notes scribbled on a piece of paper. As Dr Danielle Adams (Head of Performance Psychology at the EIS) explained, with any major event, it is common to have flashbacks of what happened. There is this whole array of things that come to your mind, which is normal, and it takes some time for the dust to settle. After the hot debrief, time zero is about being in the present moment, giving yourself permission to be present with your baby in those first moments, whilst also acknowledging that there may be waves of emotions with ups and downs, and to spend time with your support network such as family and friends. This process offers space to think about what's happened during a major event (the Olympic Games, giving birth) and to tell yourself that it is okay to experience all of these emotions.

Once the dust has settled, you may be ready to spend time trying to process the emotion. The approach the EIS takes when processing the emotion is decompression, which in our conversation Danielle explained as 'a method that is used to help athletes and coaches process their emotions, make sense of their experiences, and ultimately recover more quickly'. There are six steps to processing the emotion in this stage:

1. **Contracting**
   a. What do you want to get out of the emotional decompression?
2. **Timeline of meaningful moments**
   a. Capture the meaningful moments of the event, consider who were part of these moments, how this compared to your expectations, what did you do?
3. **Thoughts, feelings, and emotions**
   a. From the timeline, pick an event that was critical to you. Can you label the emotions (for example, 'I feel frustration when this happened', rather than 'I am frustrated'), can you label your thoughts?
      i. When thinking about these emotions, it is important to acknowledge that not everyone will react to events in the same way and that it is normal for emotions to come and go.
      ii. An 'emotion wheel' can be helpful to name emotions
   b. What impact did these thoughts or emotions have on you?
4. **Recognise impact**
   a. Looking back at those critical moments, what got you through these moments? What sticks out for you as something you did? What are the strengths that you want to keep in your toolbox?
   b. Give yourself credit for going through the experiences of the event

5. **Utilising meaning for looking ahead**
   a. Looking forward from the experience, where are you now and what is the perspective that you have now, or the meaning that you gained from the event?
      i. What do you see ahead, in the horizon? How can you use this perspective gained from the event moving forward?
      ii. What is your plan for looking after *you*?
      iii. What is something that you are looking forward to?
6. **Summarising sense-making and action points**
   a. Where do I want to go from here?
   b. What are my action points?

This structured process demonstrates the importance of giving yourself space to think about what happened without immediately jumping to evaluating outcomes. When it comes to giving birth, there is often a tendency to judge the 'performance'. What this process does is to remove you from this judgement, and instead giving you that non-judgemental space so that you can enjoy the present moment so that you can take the next step of your journey when you are ready.

As a task, when you are ready, what you could do is to draw a time-line of meaningful moments, like the one below, with as much detail as you feel like adding. You could ask yourself, when it comes to my childbirth experience, what are the things or events that happened? When did the labour experience start for you? Perhaps you start with the water breaking, or the first call to the midwife after contractions started. You can label those events with the thoughts and feelings that you recall having at this time. This timeline will give you a visual over-view of the birth experience, it helps you to validate your thoughts and feelings, and importantly it offers you the opportunity to acknowledge what is that you have been through and what you have achieved. After all, there are a lot of strengths from you having given birth that you can take with you.

Mucus plug loss
- Oh, this must be 'the bloody show', that's not that bad
- In denial, it could still take ages

Water breaking

Oh crap, the baby will come out soon. I don't really understand why these contractions don't become more regular

Abandon plan A & B
- I feel upset about the birth I won't get
- I feel angry about not being heard
- The consultant does not seem to like me
- Have we made the right decision?
- Okay well let's crack on with it and make the best of it

Final push
- This last bit of energy literally came from my toes. How on earth did I make it
- I feel proud

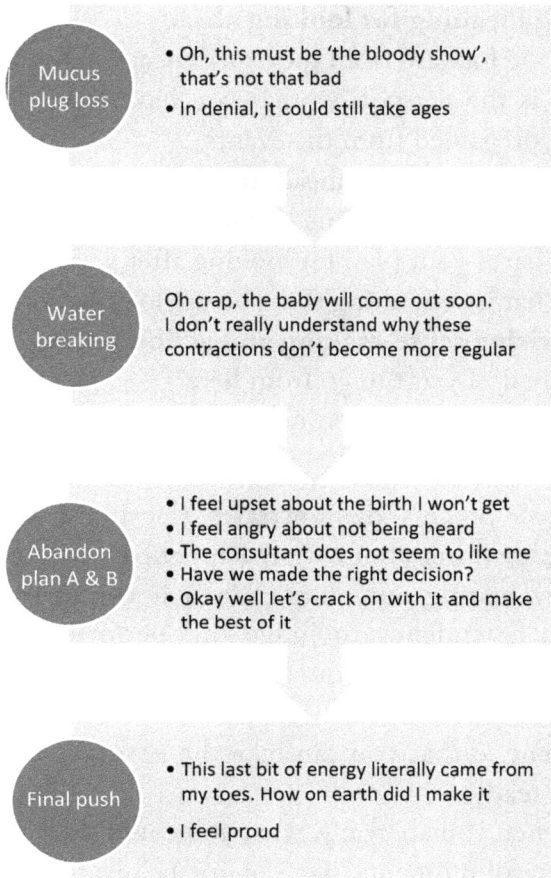

In summary, this approach that was developed by the English Institute of Sport is important to consider in relation to child birth; it's such an intense time where new mothers often feel they have very little time for themselves, and sometimes we can also be very quick to judge ourselves and our 'performance'. This process also emphasises the important role the support network can play to help you navigate the emotional rollercoaster. What is important to note is that when athletes in the English Institute of Sport process the emotion (the third stage) that this is guided by professionally trained staff. As such, you might feel that it is helpful to speak to someone with experience in psychological debriefing, especially decompressing emotions. Furthermore, you may find that from your timeline and the action points that you need some help with filling in some details to better understand what happened during your labour. This could be to arrange a meeting about what happened with someone who was there, such as a birth partner, midwife, or other health professional.

Debriefs with health professionals

It can happen that women have blocked out parts of the labour or simply don't remember aspects of their labour, which is quite normal considering everything that is going on. But for some, the experience was traumatic and blocking out memories can be an indicator of this trauma, where it can be difficult to piece together what happened. If you feel that you have experienced birth trauma, do seek help, as it can have a lasting effect on you. Often birth trauma is associated with situations where the emergency button was pushed, such as massive haemorrhaging or the baby needing to be resuscitated. It is important to remember that these situations do not always cause birth trauma. Moreover, birth trauma does not only come from those types of situations, it can be the way someone spoke to you, or you are not feeling empowered by decisions that were made, really, as Pip Davies (midwife) emphasised any aspect that felt traumatic to you, or your birth partner, can be birth trauma. Birth partners are important to consider when it comes to filling in gaps you might have when recalling your experiences, they can help you piece together what happened. Birth partners are also important to consider of being at risk of birth trauma, as the birth partner will have seen and heard everything, this can be terrifying, especially if they are not prepared for it. As such, it is important for birth partners to share their experiences with someone as well if they feel the need too, or for them to go through the stages of decompression. Let's not forget that it can also be a big event for them.

A meeting to go through your labour notes can happen many months, or even years down the line, perhaps when you are pregnant again, or if you keep having recurring dreams or thoughts about something that happened during labour and you haven't been able to decompress your emotions. One of the women I spoke with, whilst being pregnant with her second child a few years after giving birth to her first child, decided to have a debrief where she went through her hospital notes from the birth of her first child with a midwife. She experienced this process as healing and it helped her to make sense of what had happened. She felt that this gave her more confidence and ownership over the process going forward. Hospitals in the United Kingdom should offer you the opportunity for a debrief or at least give you access to your hospital notes. It is important to consider that the meeting may not be with the same person who was in the room with you. If possible, try to make sure you engage in the process when you are in a calm state and have some headspace, so that you have the opportunity to fully engage in the process. If you decide to have this meeting, asking about the 'whys' are important. Some questions you have may be about not understanding why something happened, or even though processes were explained to you, you did not take any of it in because you were overwhelmed by pain or anxiety.

Reflecting on your strengths

Throughout the book, there have been tasks that encouraged you to reflect on your experiences. Reflection is about making sense of a situation, and it is such a key tool for sports people, yet often overlooked. In the heat of the moment, it may be the last thing on someone's mind, yet reflection is one of the key stages of self-regulation and growth. It can help us move forward. When I explain self-regulation (see also chapter 1) to my students and ask them how much they engaged in reflection when they play their sports, often only a few mentioned that they did this. Similarly, athletes I worked with have also commented that they do not always engage in reflection. From these conversations, it turns out that often reflections focus on the negative experiences, and individuals tune in less to positive experiences. If you constantly relive negative experiences through reflection, then it is no surprise that you'd rather avoid this. As covered earlier in the book, it is important to start tuning in more to positive experiences as this can boost our self-belief and make this more robust, or to learn from negative experiences rather than just focusing on reliving these. Reflection also informs goal-planning for future events. Reflecting on what you achieve during the post-partum period can also help you to become aware how you are growing into being a mother of the child that has just been born and to help you notice making progress towards new goals.

In the immediate aftermath after giving birth, reflection may not be at the forefront of your mind, and you may not have the motivation and energy to do this right away. You can use this time for a 'hot debrief' as outlined earlier in this chapter. Give yourself time and engage in self-reflection when you are ready for it. In the meantime, you might want to jot down some of your thoughts or record your birth story when you are sharing this with friends or family. You'd be surprised how quickly you forget entire fragments of the birth! After an interview with one of the mothers, I revisited a text message interaction with a friend when I shared that I thought my waters had just broken. It was fascinating to recall these very 'raw' insights into the journey. You don't need to write a lengthy birth story, these snippets of information can be just as useful when engaging in reflecting on the experience later on and this can also help with decompressing your emotions.

Reflection can be done in informal ways of reflecting, such as writing notes in a diary, recording a video, drawing, or having conversations with others. You can ask questions like, 'What happened in the situation and what were the reasons for this to happen?', 'What have I taken away from the situation?', 'What am I most proud of?'. There are also more structured, systematic, ways of reflecting, like Gibbs' reflective cycle, which is something that health practitioners, like doctors, physiotherapists, nurses, midwives, and psychologists engage in.

Sometimes I also use structured reflection with athletes as it is a nice way to distance yourself from the situation and to promote learning and growth. Whatever approach you take, it is important to remember that the reflection is about *you*, it is your journey and reflecting what it is that you have experienced, considering your individual circumstances. Of course, there may be other people involved, but when it comes to reflective practice, it is about you learning and growing from the reflection.

In different parts of this book, I have referred to the strength-based approach, and now we are getting to the end of the book, it is a timely reminder to come back to this. Whilst you want to validate your thoughts and feelings, you also want to reflect on what you have achieved, what is it that you have added to your toolbox, and which existing skills and tools have you strengthened. The maternity journey comes with amazing achievements, from growing a little person inside you to giving birth, and all there is in between. It is so easy to get on with the day, especially when you are sleep-deprived, tired, and worn out. This is okay and completely normal. Yet, recalling how strong you can be is an empowering experience and can offer you reassurance in those times when you feel a bit down. Reflecting on your achievements can also make you feel more confident when you are facing a difficult situation. One of the women told me how on top of the world she felt after giving birth to her second child. Recalling those memories was a powerful experience for her as it gave her a reminder of this, and she was not the only one who felt empowered by recalling their achievements of growing and bringing a baby into the world. Chemmy recalled how powerful she felt on her maternity journey:

I had never felt more empowered as a woman than when I was pregnant. Looking down at the bump, feeling those kicks, it's absolutely surreal that your body is doing this. I did a lot of mindfulness of visualising myself with a cape, you are superhuman. This is a time that everyone understands that you are going to be the most incredible version of yourself.

It really is amazing how strong you can be, not only physically but also mentally. If you take one thing from the book, I hope that it will be this feeling of empowerment on your maternity journey. Ready, steady, baby!

Take-home message

1. Remember that pregnancy, labour, and the post-partum period are *your* journey. Giving birth is not a competition. Carve out your own path, reflect on your strengths, and use these to empower yourself to have a path you feel motivated to take and approach the maternity and post-partum journey as a positive challenge. At the same time, allow yourself time to recover emotionally and to engage with the new baby when it is there. It will take some time to get used to the 'new' you, and it's okay to give yourself that time.

2. Pace yourself, not only during pregnancy, labour, but also during the post-partum period. Allow yourself to be patient and plan for off-days. The pregnancy, labour, and post-partum period can be unpredictable and there will be quite a few 'uncontrollables'. Having an awareness that this can happen, and drawing on strategies such as motivational self-talk or acceptance can be helpful.

3. Let's go back to your toolbox. Not every tool works for every job, you want to select the tools that work and load your toolbox with those strategies that will help you. Some tools are multi-tools and work for a lot of different jobs, whereas other ones are more specialist ones. You can think about psychological strategies in a similar way; there may be some strategies that you come back to time and time again, and some others that you may only use sporadically.

4. Practice and reflect. Reading about strategies is a good start; you need to practice the strategies to know how to use them and reflect on how you could adapt a strategy to different situations. How

could a strategy that has worked well for you in sport, or other demanding settings, work for you during the maternity journey? The more you have practiced a strategy, the more accessible this strategy will be, and knowing that the strategy works for you can give you confidence and make you feel empowered. If you are unsure, or can't remember a strategy under pressure, then switch to what you know.

5. Finally, remember that you did not get to where you were in your sport or exercise journey overnight. You have made progress over time, and you can approach the maternity journey in the same way. Be proactive, believe in yourself, and focus on what's in your control on this journey.

References and further reading

If you want to learn more about the content covered in the book chapters, I have added some resources for each chapter. Some of these are books, others are research articles. You can search for these research articles on websites such as Google Scholar or use www.researchgate .net/ – which is a website where some researchers share their work.

Chapter 1. Ready, steady … Sport psychology and your maternity journey

Augoustinos, M., Walker, I., & Donaghue, N. (2014). *Social cognition: An integrated introduction.* Sage.

Buckley, S. J. (2015). Executive summary of hormonal physiology of childbearing: evidence and implications for women, babies, and maternity care. *The Journal of Perinatal Education, 24*(3), 145–153.

De Vivo, M., & Mills, H. (2021). Laying the foundation for pregnancy physical activity profiling: a framework for providing tailored physical activity advice and guidance to pregnant women. *International Journal of Environmental Research and Public Health, 18*(11), 5996.

Farley, D., Piszczek, Ł., & Bąbel, P. (2019). Why is running a marathon like giving birth? The possible role of oxytocin in the underestimation of the memory of pain induced by labor and intense exercise. *Medical Hypotheses, 128*, 86–90.

Hoffman, K. M., Trawalter, S., Axt, J. R., & Oliver, M. N. (2016). Racial bias in pain assessment and treatment recommendations, and false beliefs about biological differences between blacks and whites. *Proceedings of the National Academy of Sciences, 113*(16), 4296–4301.

Keay, N. (2022). *Hormones, health, and human potential. A guide to understanding your hormones to optimise your health and performance.* Sequoia Books.

Mangelsdorf, J. (2017). Coping with childbirth: Brain structural associations of personal growth initiative. *Frontiers in psychology, 8*, 1829.

Meddings, N. (2017). *How to Have a Baby: Mother-gathered Guidance on Birth and New Babies*. Eynham Press.

Sandars, J., Jenkins, L., Church, H., Patel, R., Rumbold, J., Maden, M., ... & Brown, J. (2022). Applying sport psychology in health professions education: A systematic review of performance mental skills training. *Medical Teacher, 44*(1), 71–78.

Sly, D., Mellalieu, S. D., & Wagstaff, C. R. (2020). "It's psychology Jim, but not as we know it!": The changing face of applied sport psychology. *Sport, Exercise, and Performance Psychology, 9*(1), 87.

Turner, M. J., Aspin, G., Didymus, F. F., Mack, R., Olusoga, P., Wood, A. G., & Bennett, R. (2020). One case, four approaches: The application of psychotherapeutic approaches in sport psychology. *The Sport Psychologist, 34*(1), 71–83.

Wagstaff, C. R., & Leach, J. (2017). The value of strength-based approaches in SERE and sport psychology. *Military Psychology, 27(2),* 65-84.

Zimmerman, B. J. (2000). Attaining self-regulation: A social cognitive perspective. In M. Boekaerts, P. Pintrich, & M. Zeidner (Eds.), *Handbook of self-regulation* (pp. 13–39). Academic press.

Chapter 2. Seeing the maternity journey as a positive challenge, not a threat

Berentson-Shaw, J., Scott, K. M., & Jose, P. E. (2009). Do self-efficacy beliefs predict the primiparous labour and birth experience? A longitudinal study. *Journal of Reproductive and Infant Psychology, 27*(4), 357–373.

Carlsson, M., Ziegert, K., & Nissen, E. (2015). The relationship between childbirth self-efficacy and aspects of well-being, birth interventions and birth outcomes. *Midwifery, 31*(10), 1000–1007.

Elliot, A. J. (2006). The hierarchical model of approach-avoidance motivation. *Motivation and Emotion, 30*(2), 111–116.

Howarth, A. M., & Swain, N. R. (2019). Skills-based childbirth preparation increases childbirth self-efficacy for first time mothers. *Midwifery, 70*, 100–105.

Jones, M., Meijen, C., McCarthy, P. J., & Sheffield, D. (2009). A theory of challenge and threat states in athletes. *International Review of Sport and Exercise Psychology, 2*(2), 161–180.

Meijen, C., Turner, M., Jones, M. V., Sheffield, D., & McCarthy, P. (2020). A theory of challenge and threat states in athletes: A revised conceptualization. *Frontiers in Psychology, 126*.

Meijen, C., Turner, M., & Jones, M. (2022). How to see pressure in sport as a challenge, not a threat. *Frontiers for Young Minds, 10*, 681496.

Skinner, E. A. (1996). A guide to constructs of control. *Journal of Personality and Social Psychology*, *71*(3), 549.

Tinti, C., Schmidt, S., & Businaro, N. (2011). Pain and emotions reported after childbirth and recalled 6 months later: the role of controllability. *Journal of Psychosomatic Obstetrics & Gynecology*, *32*(2), 98–103.

Chapter 3. Checking in with your emotions

Baron, R. S., Cusumano, M. A., Evans, D. C., Hodne, C. J., & Logan, H. (2004). The effect of desired control and anticipated control on the stress of childbirth. *Basic and Applied Social Psychology*, *26*(4), 249–261.

Benfield, R. D., Newton, E. R., Tanner, C. J., & Heitkemper, M. M. (2014). Cortisol as a biomarker of stress in term human labor: physiological and methodological issues. *Biological Research for Nursing*, *16*(1), 64–71.

Callister, L. C., Khalaf, I., Semenic, S., Kartchner, R., & Vehvilainen-Julkunen, K. (2003). The pain of childbirth: perceptions of culturally diverse women. *Pain Management Nursing*, *4*(4), 145–154.

Hall, P. J., Foster, J. W., Yount, K. M., & Jennings, B. M. (2018). Keeping it together and falling apart: Women's dynamic experience of birth. *Midwifery*, *58*, 130–136.

Hanton, S., Thomas, O., & Maynard, I. (2004). Competitive anxiety responses in the week leading up to competition: the role of intensity, direction and frequency dimensions. *Psychology of Sport and Exercise*, *5*(2), 169–181.

Hauck, Y., Fenwick, J., Downie, J., & Butt, J. (2007). The influence of childbirth expectations on Western Australian women's perceptions of their birth experience. *Midwifery*, *23*(3), 235–247.

Olza, I., Leahy-Warren, P., Benyamini, Y., Kazmierczak, M., Karlsdottir, S. I., Spyridou, A., ... & Nieuwenhuijze, M. J. (2018). Women's psychological experiences of physiological childbirth: a meta-synthesis. *BMJ Open*, *8*(10), e020347.

Preis, H., Lobel, M., & Benyamini, Y. (2019). Between expectancy and experience: testing a model of childbirth satisfaction. *Psychology of Women Quarterly*, *43*(1), 105–117.

Thies-Lagergren, L., Ólafsdóttir, Ó. Á., & Sjöblom, I. (2021). Being in charge in an encounter with extremes. A survey study on how women experience and work with labour pain in a Nordic home birth setting. *Women and Birth*, *34*(2), 122–127.

Zhang, L., Losin, E. A. R., Ashar, Y. K., Koban, L., & Wager, T. D. (2021). Gender biases in estimation of others' pain. *The Journal of Pain*, *22*(9), 1048–1059.

Chapter 4. Birth plan overboard! Goal-setting and goal-revision

Costa, S., De Gregorio, E., Zurzolo, L., Santi, G., Ciofi, E. G., Di Gruttola, F., ... & Di Fronso, S. (2022). Athletes and coaches through the COVID-19 pandemic: A qualitative view of goal management. *International Journal of Environmental Research and Public Health, 19*(9), 5085.

Gollwitzer, P. M. (1999). Implementation intentions: Strong effects of simple plans. *American Psychologist, 54*(7), 493.

Healy, L., Tincknell-Smith, A., & Ntoumanis, N. (2018). Goal setting in sport and performance. In *Oxford Research Encyclopedia of Psychology*.

Hollander, M., de Miranda, E., van Dillen, J., de Graaf, I., Vandenbussche, F., & Holten, L. (2017). Women's motivations for choosing a high risk birth setting against medical advice in the Netherlands: a qualitative analysis. *BMC Pregnancy and Childbirth, 17*(1), 1–13.

Jeong, Y. H., Healy, L. C., & McEwan, D. (2021). The application of goal setting theory to goal setting interventions in sport: A systematic review. *International Review of Sport and Exercise Psychology* (published ahead of print).

Karlsdottir, S. I., Halldorsdottir, S., & Lundgren, I. (2014). The third paradigm in labour pain preparation and management: the childbearing woman's paradigm. *Scandinavian Journal of Caring Sciences, 28*(2), 315–327.

Kingston, K. M., & Wilson, K. M. (2008). The application of goal setting in sport. In In S. Mellalieu & S. Hanton (Eds.), *Advances in applied sport psychology* (pp. 85–133). Routledge.

Quiroz, L. H., Blomquist, J. L., Macmillan, D., Mccullough, A., & Handa, V. L. (2011). Maternal goals for childbirth associated with planned vaginal and planned cesarean birth. *American Journal of Perinatology, 28*(9), 695–702.

Chapter 5. 'I could imagine the baby descending down the birth canal': Imagery as a strategy for labour and beyond

Baird, C. L., & Sands, L. (2004). A pilot study of the effectiveness of guided imagery with progressive muscle relaxation to reduce chronic pain and mobility difficulties of osteoarthritis. *Pain Management Nursing, 5*(3), 97–104.

Boryri, T., Navidian, A., & Marghzari, N. (2019). Comparison of the effect of muscle relaxation and guided imagery on happiness and fear of childbirth in primiparous women admitted to health care centers. *International Journal of Women's Health and Reproduction Sciences, 7*(4), 490–495.

Cumming, J., Cooley, S. J., Anuar, N., Kosteli, M. C., Quinton, M. L., Weibull, F., & Williams, S. E. (2017). Developing imagery ability effectively: A guide to layered stimulus response training. *Journal of Sport Psychology in Action, 8*(1), 23–33.

Gedde-Dahl, M., & Fors, E. A. (2012). Impact of self-administered relaxation and guided imagery techniques during final trimester and birth. *Complementary Therapies in Clinical Practice, 18*(1), 60–65.

Rhodes, J., & May, J. (2021). Applied imagery for motivation: a person-centred model. *International Journal of Sport and Exercise Psychology*, 1–20.

Ryan, R. M., & Deci, E. L. (2000). Intrinsic and extrinsic motivations: Classic definitions and new directions. *Contemporary Educational Psychology, 25*(1), 54–67.

Migliorini, L., Cardinali, P., & Rania, N. (2019). How could self-determination theory be useful for facing health innovation challenges?. *Frontiers in Psychology, 10*, 1870.

Vealey, R. S., & Forlenza, S. T. (2014). Understanding and using imagery in sport. In J. M. Williams & V. Krane (Eds.), *Applied sport psychology: Personal growth to peak performance* (pp. 240–273). New York, NY: McGraw-Hill.

Chapter 6: 'I got this': Self-talk as a strategy in your toolkit

Ellis., A. (1994). The sport of avoiding sports and exercise: A rational emotive behavior therapy perspective. *The Sport Psychologist, 8*, 248–261

Fritsch, J., Feil, K., Jekauc, D., Latinjak, A. T., & Hatzigeorgiadis, A. (2022). The relationship between self-talk and affective processes in sports: a scoping review. *International Review of Sport and Exercise Psychology*, 1–34.

Furman, C. R., Kross, E., & Gearhardt, A. N. (2020). Distanced self-talk enhances goal pursuit to eat healthier. *Clinical Psychological Science, 8*(2), 366–373.

McCormick, A., & Hatzigeorgiadis, A. (2019). Self-talk and endurance performance. In C. Meijen (Ed.), *Endurance performance in sport: Psychological theory and interventions* (pp. 153–167). Routledge.

Latinjak, A. T., Hatzigeorgiadis, A., Comoutos, N., & Hardy, J. (2019). Speaking clearly... 10 years on: The case for an integrative perspective of self-talk in sport. *Sport, Exercise, and Performance Psychology, 8*(4), 353.

Turner, M. (2023). *The rational practitioner: The sport and performance psychologist's guide to practicing rational emotive behaviour therapy*. Routledge.

Turner, M., & Bennett, R. (2017). *Rational emotive behavior therapy in sport and exercise*. Routledge.

Chapter 7: The power of the breath: Breathing and mindfulness-based strategies

British Lung Foundation (2021). *How your lungs work [Brochure].* blf.org.uk/how -your-lungs-work

Duncan, L. G., & Shaddix, C. (2015). Mindfulness-based childbirth and parenting (MBCP): innovation in birth preparation to support healthy, happy families. *International Journal of Birth and Parent Education, 2*(2), 30.

Harris, R. (2019). *ACT made simple: An easy-to-read primer on acceptance and commitment therapy.* New Harbinger Publications.

Henriksen, K., Hansen, J., & Larsen, C. H. (2019). *Mindfulness and acceptance in sport: How to help athletes perform and thrive under pressure.* Routledge.

Lane, M., Morosky, C., & West, A. M. (2021). Mindfulness-Based interventions and their application to the pregnant population. *Topics in Obstetrics & Gynecology, 41*(2), 1–7.

LoMauro, A., & Aliverti, A. (2015). Respiratory physiology of pregnancy: physiology masterclass. *Breathe, 11*(4), 297-301.

Lothian, J. A. (2011). Lamaze breathing: what every pregnant woman needs to know. *The Journal of Perinatal Education, 20*(2), 118–120.

Martin, M., Seppa, M., Lehtinen, P., & Toro , T. (2016). *Breathing as a tool for self-regulation and self-reflection.* Karnac Books Ltd.

Veringa-Skiba, I. K., de Bruin, E. I., van Steensel, F. J., & Bögels, S. M. (2022). Fear of childbirth, nonurgent obstetric interventions, and newborn outcomes: A randomized controlled trial comparing mindfulness-based childbirth and parenting with enhanced care as usual. *Birth, 49*(1), 40–51.

Warriner, S., Crane, C., Dymond, M., & Krusche, A. (2018). An evaluation of mindfulness-based childbirth and parenting courses for pregnant women and prospective fathers/partners within the UK NHS (MBCP-4-NHS). *Midwifery, 64*, 1–10.

Wrønding, T., Argyraki, A., Petersen, J. F., Topsøe, M. F., Petersen, P. M., & Løkkegaard, E. C. (2019). The aesthetic nature of the birthing room environment may alter the need for obstetrical interventions–an observational retrospective cohort study. *Scientific Reports, 9*(1), 1–7.

Chapter 8: Focus: Being in the moment and letting go of the uncontrollables

Bonk, D., & Tamminen, K. A. (2022). Athletes' perspectives of preparation strategies in open-skill sports. *Journal of Applied Sport Psychology, 34*(4), 825–845.

Cotterill, S. (2015). Preparing for performance: strategies adopted across performance domains. *The Sport Psychologist, 29*(2), 158–170.

Cotterill, S. (2010). Pre-performance routines in sport: Current understanding and future directions. *International Review of Sport and Exercise Psychology, 3*(2), 132–153.

Hagan Jnr, J. E., & Schack, T. (2019). Integrating pre-game rituals and pre-performance routines in a culture-specific context: Implications for sport psychology consultancy. *International Journal of Sport and Exercise Psychology, 17*(1), 18–31.

Lidor, R., Hackfort, D., & Shack, T. (2014). Performance routines in sport: Meaning and practice. In In A. Papaioannou & D. Hackfort (Eds.), *Routledge companion to sport and exercise psychology: Global perspectives and fundamental concepts* (pp. 480–494). Routledge.

Moran, A. (2009). Attention in sport. In S. Mellalieu & S. Hanton (Eds.), *Advances in applied sport psychology: A review* (pp. 195–220). Routledge.

Moran, A. (2012). Thinking in action: Some insights from cognitive sport psychology. *Thinking Skills and Creativity, 7*(2), 85–92.

Schuijers, R. (2018). *Focus: Beter presteren door cirkeltraining* (in Dutch). Dam Uitgeverij.

Williams, J. M., Nideffer, R. M., Wilson, V. E., Sagal, M. S., & Peper, E. (2010). Concentration and strategies for controlling it. In J. M. Williams (Ed.), *Applied sport psychology: Personal growth to peak performance* (pp. 336–358). McGraw-Hill.

Chapter 9: The team behind the team: Engaging your support network

Coughlan, R., & Jung, K. E. (2005). New mothers' experiences of agency during prenatal and delivery care: clinical practice, communication and embodiment. *Journal of Prenatal & Perinatal Psychology & Health, 20*(2), 99.

Hollander, M., de Miranda, E., Smit, A. M., de Graaf, I., Vandenbussche, F., van Dillen, J., & Holten, L. (2020). 'She convinced me'-partner involvement in choosing a high risk birth setting against medical advice in the Netherlands: a qualitative analysis. *PloS One, 15*(2), e0229069.

Leap, N., & Hunter, B. (2016). *Supporting women for labour and birth: A thoughtful guide*. Routledge.

Lunda, P., Minnie, C. S., & Benadé, P. (2018). Women's experiences of continuous support during childbirth: a meta-synthesis. *BMC Pregnancy and Childbirth, 18*(1), 1–11.

Olza, I., Leahy-Warren, P., Benyamini, Y., Kazmierczak, M., Karlsdottir, S. I., Spyridou, A., ... & Nieuwenhuijze, M. J. (2018). Women's psychological experiences of physiological childbirth: a meta-synthesis. *BMJ Open, 8*(10).

Mgawadere, F., Smith, H., Asfaw, A., Lambert, J., & van den Broek, N. (2019). "There is no time for knowing each other": Quality of care during childbirth in a low resource setting. *Midwifery, 75*, 33–40.

Sargent, C., & Stark, N. (1989). Childbirth education and childbirth models: parental perspectives on control, anesthesia, and technological intervention in the birth process. *Medical Anthropology Quarterly, 3*(1), 36–51.

Van Vulpen, M., Heideveld-Gerritsen, M., van Dillen, J., Maatman, S. O., Ockhuijsen, H., & van den Hoogen, A. (2021). First-time fathers' experiences and needs during childbirth: A systematic review. *Midwifery, 94*, 102921.

Chapter 10: Bringing it home: The post-partum period

Callister, L. C. (2004). Making meaning: Women's birth narratives. *Journal of Obstetric, Gynecologic, & Neonatal Nursing, 33*(4), 508–518.

Callister, L. C., Khalaf, I., Semenic, S., Kartchner, R., & Vehvilainen-Julkunen, K. (2003). The pain of childbirth: perceptions of culturally diverse women. *Pain Management Nursing, 4*(4), 145–154.

Carter, S. K. (2010). Beyond control: body and self in women's childbearing narratives. *Sociology of Health & Illness, 32*(7), 993–1009.

Chow, G. M., & Luzzeri, M. (2019). Post-event reflection: a tool to facilitate self-awareness, self-monitoring, and self-regulation in athletes. *Journal of Sport Psychology in Action, 10*(2), 106–118.

Donnelly, G. M., Rankin, A., Mills, H., Marlize, D. E., Goom, T. S., & Brockwell, E. (2020). Infographic. guidance for medical, health and fitness professionals to support women in returning to running postnatally. *British Journal of Sports Medicine, 54*(18), 1114–1115.

English Institute of Sport (2021). Performance decompression: Post-games celebration and support https://eis2win.co.uk/article/performance -decompression-post-games-celebration-and-support

Harvey, J., Pearson, E. S., Mantler, T., & Gotwals, J. K. (2020). 'Be kind to yourself–because you're doing fine': using self-determination theory to explore the health-related experiences of primiparous women participating in a co-active life coaching intervention. *Coaching: An International Journal of Theory, Research and Practice, 13*(1), 78–91.

Hoogenboom, M. (2022). *The motherhood complex: The story of our changing selves.* Little, Brown Book Group.

Kinchin, D. (2007). *A guide to psychological debriefing: Managing emotional decompression and post-traumatic stress disorder.* Jessica Kingsley Publishers.

Lundgren, I. (2005). Swedish women's experience of childbirth 2 years after birth. *Midwifery, 21*(4), 346–354.

Massey, K. L., & Whitehead, A. E. (2022). Pregnancy and motherhood in elite sport: The longitudinal experiences of two elite athletes. *Psychology of Sport and Exercise, 60.*

Negron, R., Martin, A., Almog, M., Balbierz, A., & Howell, E. A. (2013). Social support during the postpartum period: mothers' views on needs, expectations, and mobilization of support. *Maternal and Child Health Journal, 17*(4), 616–623.

Richards, D. P. (2020). The patient as person: an update. *British Journal of Sports Medicine, 54*(23), 1376–1376.

APPENDIX

Gibbs' reflective cycle

In chapter 10, I briefly referred to Gibb's reflective cycle as a more structured approach to reflection. It is designed to be a step-by-step approach to help you make sense of an experience, and it is often used in healthcare settings as a way to learn and develop. You can use this structured reflection to reflect on your labour, experiences during the post-partum journey (perhaps getting back to training) and so on. Remember that you don't just need to reflect on situations that you feel are 'negative', you can learn just as much from situations that you felt went well. There are six steps that you follow, which I have described below, with a few questions that you can ask yourself for each step

	Questions that can help with the reflection
1. Description – Recall the situation	What happened? Where was it? When was it? Who were there?
	What did everyone, including me, do?
	Why was I there?
	What was the outcome?
2. Feelings – Recall the feelings and the thoughts I had in the situation	What did I feel before, during, after?
	What did I think before, during, after?
	What do I think others in the situations may have felt or thought?
	What do I feel/think about it now?
3. Evaluation – Consider the positive and negative outcomes of the situation	What worked well in the situation?
	What did not go so well?
	What was positive?
	What was negative?

(Continued)

(Continued)

	Questions that can help with the reflection
4. Analysis – Consider the evidence	Why did it go well? Why did it not go well? What was it that you did and what was it that other people did in the situation that made it positive and/or negative? What do I need to help better understand the situation?
5. Conclusion – Consider what have I learned	What did I take away from the situation? How could I turn it into a positive challenge? What are other things I could have done? What skills (such as coping strategies) could I work on to help me in similar situations?
6. Action plan – Consider what to do the next time	What will I do a next time? What can I do to develop the skill or coping strategies for this situation? What help do I need?

www.ingramcontent.com/pod-product-compliance
Lightning Source LLC
Chambersburg PA
CBHW071412210326
41597CB00020B/3465